LIVING YOUNG

Biohacking Techniques and Exercises to Improve Your Lifespan

Lara Hemeryck, PhD
and Anastasia Mabel

Foreword by **Sergey Young**
FOUNDER OF BOLD LONGEVITY GROWTH FUND

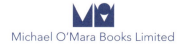

Michael O'Mara Books Limited

First published in Great Britain in 2025 by
Michael O'Mara Books Limited
9 Lion Yard
Tremadoc Road
London SW4 7NQ

EU representative:
Authorised Rep Compliance Ltd
Ground Floor
71 Baggot Street Lower
Dublin D02 P593
Ireland

This product is made of material from well-
managed, FSC®-certified forests and other
controlled sources. The manufacturing processes
conform to the environmental regulations of the
country of origin.

For further information see www.mombooks.
com/about/sustainability-climate-focus

Report any safety issues to product.safety@
mombooks.com and see www.mombooks.com/
contact/product-safety

UK edition:
ISBN: 978-1-78929-742-3 in paperback print
    format
ISBN: 978-1-78929-839-0 in ebook format

US edition:
ISBN: 978-1-78929-798-0 in paperback print
    format
ISBN: 978-1-78929-812-3 in ebook format

1 2 3 4 5 6 7 8 9 10

The information provided in this book is intended
for general informational and educational purposes
only and is not a substitute for professional
medical advice, diagnosis or treatment. Always
seek the advice of your doctor or other qualified
health provider with any questions you may have
regarding a medical condition or health objective.
Neither the publisher nor the author can accept
any liability for any injury or loss that may occur as
a result of information given in this book.

Cover design by Ana Bjezancevic
and Barbara Ward
Designed and typeset by Claire Cater and
Barbara Ward
Printed and bound in China

www.mombooks.com

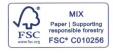

MIX
Paper | Supporting
responsible forestry
FSC® C010256

LIVING
YOUNG

CONTENTS

FOREWORD

We are standing on the threshold of one of the most remarkable moments in human history. For centuries, we have been fascinated by the mystery of ageing – why it happens, how it affects us and whether it can be slowed or even reversed. Today, we are closer than ever to cracking the code of human biology. Advances in artificial intelligence and computing power are enabling scientists to analyze vast datasets and detect patterns that have previously been invisible. In the next ten years, these advances will help us find solutions to ageing and age-related diseases, giving us a wealth of choice on how to grow young. Over the next twenty years, other breakthrough technologies – such as gene editing and gene therapy, organ regeneration and longevity-in-a-pill – will revolutionize health and extend life in ways we once only dreamed of.

But here is the question: why wait?

We already have the tools to transform our health and wellbeing – *today*. Science has repeatedly confirmed that the lifestyle choices we make – how we eat, move, sleep, think and live – have the power to add five to ten happy and healthy years to our lives. We don't need to wait for cutting-edge technology to emerge; we can begin our longevity journey right now, with simple, everyday habits that enable us to maintain optimal vitality and experience more vibrant lives.

This is what makes this book so special: it is a guide to the exciting world of longevity science, distilling decades of research into clear, actionable advice for anyone looking to take control of their health. Whether you are completely new to the concept of longevity or are already exploring ways to optimize your wellbeing, this book provides a practical roadmap. It is not just about living longer, it is about being healthier and happier at any age.

What sets this book apart is its simplicity. Longevity is a complex subject, but here it is broken down into manageable and engaging sections, covering the core pillars of a healthy life: diet, exercise, sleep, brain health and purpose. These are not abstract ideas: you will be given actionable tools that you can start using immediately. Moreover, this book does not require you to overhaul your entire life overnight, nor adhere to extreme practices. Instead, it offers practical tips that are easy to understand and incorporate into your daily routine. It recognizes that longevity is not just about science and technology, it is also about the choices we make every day, the habits we build and the mindset we cultivate.

So, as you begin this journey, know that you are stepping into a future full of promise. You will find that you already have the tools, knowledge and ability to lead a life that is not only long but also healthy, happy and fulfilling. This book will be your trusted companion along the way.

Happy reading – and happy living!

Sergey Young
Co-founder, BOLD Longevity Growth Fund
Author, *The Science and Technology of Growing Young*

'You'll never change your life until you change something you do daily.'

John C. Maxwell

Author, speaker and leadership coach

INTRODUCTION

Many people think longevity is a matter of luck or good genes. But what if it's not just inherited but something you can actively engineer?

Studies show that only 20–25 per cent of your longevity is shaped by genetics. The rest is influenced by your daily habits, actions, thoughts and even your social connections. That means you have real control over how you age and how you feel along the way. This book gives you simple, practical strategies to support your body, build up your energy and help you feel younger – starting today.

Living Young is not about chasing immortality or perfection. It's about truly *enjoying* your years, not just adding more of them to your lifespan. It's about staying connected to yourself, to others and to what matters most to you. And it's about creating a lifestyle that supports your health, energy and joy, no matter your age.

What follows are five life-changing pillars for longevity: how to eat, move, sleep, think and live, to slow down ageing and help you feel your best. All you need to do is start!

EAT: NOURISHING FOR LONGEVITY

In the Eat chapter, we'll explore what foods support your energy, DNA repair, detoxification and brain health. We'll also cover how to find the right balance of protein, fats and carbs. Moreover, together we will decide whether alcohol and caffeine can be part of a longevity-friendly diet.

MOVE: THE POWER OF EXERCISE

In the Move chapter, we'll look beyond traditional exercise routines to explore how daily movement can be seamlessly integrated into your life. From walking and strength training to yoga and Qigong, the goal is to find activities that you enjoy and can sustain. We'll also examine the science behind exercise and ageing, exploring how movement stimulates brain health, reduces the risk of chronic diseases and enhances overall wellbeing.

SLEEP: RESTORING THE MIND AND BODY

Sleep is when your body repairs itself – from cellular regeneration to hormone regulation, to memory consolidation. We'll dive into what it truly means to sleep well, how to sync up with your circadian rhythm and how to identify your chronotype. You'll get simple, practical strategies to create an environment and routine that makes great sleep your default.

THINK: KEEPING
THE BRAIN SHARP

The Think chapter explores the powerful connection between brain health, stress and mindset. You'll discover how chronic stress can accelerate ageing – and how mindfulness, continuous learning and emotional awareness can protect both your brain and your body. We'll share practical tools to help you build a more resilient mind, rewire unhelpful habits and stay mentally agile for decades to come.

LIVE: FINDING YOUR PURPOSE

Here, we zoom out and ask: what's it all for? Research shows that having a sense of purpose is one of the most powerful predictors of longevity. In this chapter, we'll help you discover what purpose means to you – whether through creativity, community, caretaking or connection. Whether it's a pet, a partner or a bigger mission, we'll explore how meaning supports both your mental and your physical health.

As you begin this journey, remember: it's not about chasing perfect health – it's about creating a life that supports the person you want to become at forty, sixty, eighty and beyond. Small, consistent choices can lead to extraordinary change. Because longevity isn't just about how long you live, it's about how alive you *feel* while you're living. Let's keep you living young!

'Let food be thy medicine and medicine be thy food.'

Hippocrates

Ancient Greek physician and philosopher

EAT

There's a reason so many breakthroughs in health and longevity research point back to food. Nutrition isn't just fuel – it's biological information. Every bite sends molecular signals that can influence gene expression, shape your gut microbiome, regulate inflammation and even signal to your cells how fast (or how slow) to age. Your plate is one of the most powerful levers you can pull to influence your healthspan and lifespan.

Research consistently shows that what we eat plays a direct role in how long and how well we live. One such study has demonstrated that switching from a standard Western diet to a nutrient-dense, whole-foods-based diet may add up to ten years to your lifespan. The best news? It is never too late to start. Even at age seventy, adopting certain dietary habits can add four to five more vibrant years – not just in lifespan but in healthspan too.

With all the noise about 'healthy diets' – paleo, keto, vegan, intermittent fasting, low FODMAP – it's easy to feel overwhelmed. But one way of eating continues to rise to the top: nutrient-dense whole-food diets such as the Mediterranean diet. Backed by decades of research, it's been shown to reduce the risk of all-cause mortality, heart disease and cognitive decline.

In one study of over 25,000 women, better adherence to the Mediterranean diet was associated with a 23 per cent lower risk of dying from any cause.

THE MEDITERRANEAN DIET

The Mediterranean diet is the way people from countries bordering the Mediterranean Sea (particularly Greece, Italy and Spain) tend to eat. It consists of whole, minimally processed foods such as fruits, vegetables, healthy fats, whole grains, nuts, legumes, fish and meat. People who eat the Mediterranean way don't tend to diet or count calories to stay lean and healthy – they simply eat whole foods each day. The next few pages will discuss the key components of the Mediterranean diet.

HEALTHY FATS

For decades, fats were vilified. But stripping fat from our food didn't make us healthier: it actually .made us sicker. The real argument shouldn't be whether to have fat or avoid it, but rather what *type* of fat we eat.

The Mediterranean diet features a generous intake of monounsaturated fats (like those in extra virgin olive oil) and omega-3 polyunsaturated fats from fatty fish and walnuts. These fats help modulate gene expression tied to inflammation and metabolism, improve insulin sensitivity and support hormone production and brain cell membrane integrity. In fact, when healthy fats made up around 35 per cent of a lower-calorie diet, they were shown to support sustained weight loss versus a low-fat diet – meaning there's no need to fear foods like olive oil, avocado, fatty fish, nuts and seeds.

When it comes to fats, quality matters just as much as quantity. Processing, high heat and additives can strip nutrients and create inflammatory byproducts that are linked to heart disease, obesity and chronic inflammation.

Stick with extra virgin olive oil for salads or stovetop cooking – yes, even at higher temperatures. Despite common myths, high-quality extra virgin olive oil has a relatively stable smoke point up to 205°C / 400°F and retains many of its benefits when heated. Just make sure it comes in a dark glass bottle, which helps protect the delicate polyphenols from light damage. For very high-heat cooking, coconut oil is a solid alternative due to its oxidative stability.

And most importantly: ditch all highly processed industrial seed oils like canola, corn, soybean, safflower, and sunflower oil, also often added to many highly-processed foods.

MEAT AND FISH

Red meat is a great source of iron and vitamin B12, both nutrients that become especially important as we age. When possible, choose organic, grass-fed and pasture-raised options for higher nutrient quality and fewer unwanted additives, but don't let perfection be a barrier. Poultry is a leaner protein choice and provides B-vitamins, zinc and selenium, which are crucial for energy production, immune function and metabolic health. Choosing skin-on, bone-in poultry offers added nutritional value thanks to the connective tissue, collagen and minerals that support joint, skin and overall health.

Fish, especially fatty fish such as salmon, sardines and mackerel, should be a staple. These types of fish are rich in omega-3 fatty acids, which help reduce inflammation and lower blood pressure – two critical factors in preventing heart disease. Opt for wild-caught fish whenever possible, as it tends to have lower levels of contaminants like pesticides and antibiotics compared to farmed fish.

WHOLE GRAINS

Whole grains like oats, barley, brown rice and whole wheat can be nutritional powerhouses. They're rich in fibre, vitamins and minerals – and that fibre does more than just aid digestion. It binds to cholesterol in your digestive system, helping to clear out excess cholesterol. The fibre and prebiotics in whole grains also nourish the beneficial bacteria in your gut, supporting a healthier microbiome and smoother digestion. Whole grains also help promote satiety and provide sustained energy throughout the day. That said, whole grains are still high in carbohydrates, which convert to glucose in our bodies and may raise our blood sugar levels.

Refined grains such as pasta and white bread have been stripped of their fibre and essential nutrients. They can cause even sharper blood sugar spikes, which over time may contribute to type 2 diabetes and obesity. If you do choose to eat them, pair them with fibre- and protein-rich foods to help blunt the blood sugar response.

PLANTS

Fresh, seasonal fruits and vegetables are the foundation – not side dishes – of a Mediterranean plate. The impact of these foods goes far beyond fibre and vitamins. The natural pigments (known as phytonutrients) that give plants their vibrant colours act as powerful signalling molecules. They interact with our genes, support mitochondrial function (the energy generators inside each cell that power everything from thinking to healing) and influence key inflammatory pathways.

Beta-carotene, found in orange carrots and sweet potatoes, converts to vitamin A in our bodies and supports immune function, as well as skin and eye health, reducing the risk of age-related macular degeneration of the eye by 25 per cent.

Nitrate in leafy greens such as kale and spinach enhances nitric oxide production, which improves blood flow and reduces blood pressure and the risk of heart disease.

The phytonutrient lycopene, which gives beetroot, watermelons and tomatoes their red colour, may help prevent certain cancers and neurodegenerative diseases such as Alzheimer's. Cooking tomatoes helps make lycopene more bioavailable, and consuming them with a healthy fat source, like olive oil, further enhances lycopene absorption.

When purchasing plants, shopping locally and seasonally helps ensure your produce will be nutritionally superior.

It's worth noting that while a high intake of fibrous vegetables supports long-term metabolic and microbiome health, it may temporarily irritate the gut lining in those with compromised digestion – which is estimated to affect 40 per cent of the global population. In these cases, a short-term elimination or gut-repair approach may be necessary to reduce inflammation and rebuild digestive resilience before expanding into a high-fibre diet.

LEGUMES AND NUTS

Legumes such as beans, lentils and chickpeas are deeply nourishing. They are packed with fibre, minerals and plant-based protein, and they release energy slowly thanks to their low glycaemic index. This makes them ideal for supporting stable blood sugar and long-lasting fullness. In some meals, they can even replace grains entirely.

Nuts and seeds are equally impressive. Varieties like almonds, walnuts and chia seeds offer heart-healthy fats, brain-boosting antioxidants and essential nutrients like magnesium. They've been linked to reduced inflammation and a lower risk of heart disease and certain cancers. Try eating them at the end of your meal, when you've already satisfied your hunger, to avoid over-snacking without missing out on their benefits.

DAIRY

Dairy is one of the most debated topics in nutrition, and for good reason. Up to 70 per cent of adults worldwide have some degree of lactose intolerance, and for others the issue isn't lactose but the type of casein protein (A1 beta-casein) that causes bloating, fatigue, joint pain or skin issues.

For those who tolerate it, high-quality dairy that's organic or pasture-raised can offer protein, calcium, B12 and probiotics, especially from fermented options like kefir, yoghurt or aged cheese. If dairy has previously caused issues, try A2 milk (which is easier to digest for many) or goat or sheep's milk.

On the surface, the Mediterranean diet is about food – but at its heart, it's about connection, presence and prevention. Food is information. Every bite speaks to your genes.

ELIMINATE ALLERGENS AND FOOD SENSITIVITIES

Chronic inflammation is a silent driver of ageing and disease, and for many people, undetected food allergies or sensitivities are a major contributor. Conditions like heart disease, diabetes, autoimmune disorders and gut dysfunction have all been linked to long-term inflammatory responses triggered by what we eat. Two of the most common culprits? Dairy and gluten. While both can be beneficial additions to a low-inflammatory and high-quality diet, they may not be right for you – especially if you notice symptoms like bloating, fatigue, skin issues or brain fog after eating them.

Food allergies are immune responses that can cause serious reactions like hives, swelling or difficulty breathing and require immediate medical attention. To test for allergies, doctors may use skin prick testing (to test for immediate reactions) or ELISA blood testing to measure antibody responses to foods. These tests can be helpful, but they aren't perfect – false positives are common, especially in cases of sensitization – where the immune system reacts to a food, even without symptoms.

Food intolerances occur when the body can't properly digest certain foods – like in lactose or histamine intolerance – and don't involve the immune system. Food sensitivities, on the other hand, often trigger delayed immune responses that can lead to symptoms like bloating, fatigue or joint pain. A compromised gut barrier – commonly referred to as 'leaky gut' – can blur the line between these conditions, allowing more food particles to interact with the immune system and potentially trigger chronic inflammation.

For sensitivities and intolerances, testing is less reliable. The best approach is thought to be an elimination diet: remove the most likely triggers (e.g. gluten, dairy, eggs) for two to four weeks, then reintroduce them one by one and observe how your body reacts. If symptoms return, eliminate the offending food for another six months before testing again. If symptoms persist after reintroduction, keep the food out for longer, typically another three to six months, before trying to reintroduce again.

You may want to keep a daily diary of symptoms, especially during the re-introduction phase. While the elimination diet can be done on your own, carry it out under medical supervision for best results.

Testing should always be done in a clinical setting, especially for allergies. Be cautious with popular at-home food sensitivity tests that measure IgG antibodies – these reflect exposure, not intolerance or sensitivity. IgG is a memory antibody, so a high result often just means you've eaten that food recently, not that it's necessarily causing harm.

MASTER YOUR GLUCOSE: FIND THE CARBS THAT WORK FOR YOU

Carbohydrates are one of the most debated macronutrients in longevity science – and also one of the most individual. The real question isn't how many carbs you eat but how well your body manages the glucose they produce.

If you're curious about your personal 'carb sweet spot', try tracking how different meals affect your energy, mood and cravings. Tools like a continuous glucose monitor (CGM), glucometer, or a simple food and mood journal can reveal helpful patterns – like which carbs keep you feeling steady and which might cause crashes or cravings. Working with a healthcare provider to assess markers like fasting glucose, HbA1c or post-meal blood sugar can offer even deeper insights into how your body processes carbohydrates so you can tailor your plate with concrete blood test results, rather than blind guesswork.

SUPPORT HEALTHY GLUCOSE LEVELS

Your body breaks down all carbohydrates into glucose, the sugar your cells use for energy. But not all carbs affect blood sugar the same way, and how your body handles glucose can make a big difference in how you feel day to day.

Instead of obsessing over grams or cutting carbs altogether, focus on how to stabilize blood sugar and avoid sharp spikes that can lead to crashes, cravings and fatigue. Many of the practical tips over the next few pages have been popularized by biochemist Jessie Inchauspé, also known as the Glucose Goddess, whose work has helped millions understand how food order and pairing impact glucose. These strategies are grounded in science and easy to implement:

- Start your day with protein. A high-protein, low-sugar breakfast (think eggs, Greek yoghurt or lentils with greens) sets the tone for stable energy and appetite regulation.

- Use food pairing to your advantage. Combine carbs with protein, fat or fibre to slow glucose absorption. For example, pair fruit with nuts or eat veggies before starches.

- Move after meals. A ten- to twenty-minute walk or even a few squats can significantly lower your post-meal blood sugar by increasing glucose uptake in your muscles.

- Try apple cider vinegar. Taking 1–2 teaspoons diluted in water before a high-carb meal may blunt post-meal glucose spikes thanks to its acetic acid content.

So, should you just go low-carb? Low-carb diets like keto and Atkins often promise quick results – and for good reason. By dramatically lowering glucose intake, they can reduce hunger, stabilize energy and lead to rapid fat loss. In clinical settings, ketogenic diets have even shown promise for managing epilepsy, brain trauma, certain cancers and metabolic disease.

But there's a catch: the quality of your fats and proteins matters. Many popular low-carb plans rely on high intakes of processed meats and saturated fats, without enough fibre or micronutrients. This imbalance may explain why long-term adherence to low-carb diets – especially when heavy on animal products – has been linked to increased risk of premature death, according to research published in the *Lancet*.

And just as importantly: keto is not universally ideal. Some people thrive with more carbohydrates in their diet, particularly those who are physically active, menstruating or experiencing signs of sluggish thyroid or adrenal function. Others may benefit from moderate carb restriction if they have insulin resistance, PCOS or blood sugar instability. Your metabolic flexibility, hormone status and even liver function can all influence how well you tolerate different macronutrient patterns. If a low-carb or keto diet leaves you feeling fatigued, constipated, anxious or with disrupted sleep or cycles, it may be a sign that your body needs more carbs, not fewer.

Rather than jumping to extremes, a better approach is to focus on quality first, then use tools like symptom tracking, blood glucose monitoring and lab testing to personalize your intake. Find the level of carbs that supports your energy, metabolism and long-term health.

POWER UP WITH PROTEIN

Protein is the building block of your body. It's important for maintaining muscle mass, repairing tissues, making hormones and supporting metabolic health. As you get older, protein becomes even more important, particularly to prevent muscle loss (a condition known as sarcopenia), which can lead to frailty and reduced mobility. Maintaining muscle also plays a key role in regulating metabolism and maintaining a healthy weight.

How much protein do we need? While the baseline recommendation is around 0.8 grams of protein per kilogram of body weight per day, research now shows that adults over thirty need to consume slightly more – often 1.2–2.0 grams per kilogram per day. This generally works out to be about 25–30 grams of protein per meal. The exact amount depends on your lifestyle. If you're strength training, recovering from stress or transitioning away from a high-sugar diet, protein plays an even bigger role. It helps regulate appetite, supports stable blood sugar and makes it easier to feel satisfied after meals.

When it comes to quality, not all proteins are created equal. Animal proteins (such as eggs, fish, poultry, red meat and dairy) contain all essential amino acids in forms that are more easily absorbed and used by the body. They also provide key nutrients like vitamin B12, iron and bioavailable zinc, which are very hard to get in sufficient quantities from plant sources and are important for hormone production, detoxification and energy. Plant-based proteins (like lentils, beans, quinoa, tofu, nuts and seeds) can still play a valuable role, especially when eaten in variety. But gram for gram, they're less concentrated in protein and often come with higher amounts of carbohydrates or fat. For example, nuts and nut butters are frequently marketed as high-protein snacks, but they're primarily sources of fat, not protein. It would take a large amount of nuts to meet the same protein target you'd hit with a modest portion of chicken or fish.

If you follow a vegetarian or vegan diet, focus on diversity. Combine legumes, whole grains, beans and soy-based foods across your meal to cover your essential amino acids over the course of the day. While some plants are lower in certain essential amino acids, this doesn't mean you need to combine them perfectly at every meal. Your body pools amino acids over the day, so eating a variety of plant foods across your meals will cover your needs just fine.

Including a quality protein source at each meal is one of the simplest ways to support blood sugar balance, help with appetite and weight regulation, and make meals more satiating.

INCLUDE METHYL-RICH FOODS

Methylation is a mechanism of epigenetic expression, which refers to how genes are turned on or off (meaning whether a gene is actively used by the body or remains inactive). This process plays a key role in DNA repair, energy production, detoxification and even the synthesis of neurotransmitters.

However, approximately 40 per cent of the global population has at least one variant of the MTHFR (methylenetetrahydrofolate reductase) gene mutation, which can slow down or impair the methylation process. An MTHFR gene variation can make it harder for the body to process folate, a B-vitamin, leading to potential issues with energy, mood and heart health. The MTHFR gene codes for an enzyme that helps the body process folate and convert it into its active, usable form. This enzyme is essential for producing glutathione, processing hormones, detoxifying properly and maintaining cardiovascular and neurological health. When there's a mutation or variant in this gene, your body may struggle to metabolize folate, detox efficiently or maintain balanced neurotransmitters – impacting energy, mood, fertility and more.

Genetic testing for the MTHFR gene is available from private laboratories if you'd like to know your status and understand how it might affect your health, allowing you to tailor your diet and take supplements to meet your individual needs.

Beyond your genetics, incorporating foods rich in methyl groups can help boost the methylation process and promote overall longevity. Frequently include methylation-donor foods such as beetroot, shiitake mushrooms, dark leafy greens and cruciferous vegetables such as broccoli, cauliflower and kale. These foods will act like fuel for your body's repair and renewal systems, which everyone can benefit from.

AVOID PROCESSED FOODS AND ADDED SUGARS

Processed foods and added sugars are some of the most harmful offenders in today's diet. They are linked to inflammation, cardiovascular disease and a host of metabolic diseases including obesity, insulin resistance and type 2 diabetes, the latter being the eighth leading cause of death in the world. Furthermore, research has shown that excess added sugar can make our cells age faster. This includes our skin – added sugar can cause it to wrinkle.

As such, reducing your intake of processed foods and added sugars can not only significantly lower your risk of life-threatening diseases and help maintain better overall health, but even slow down the visible signs of ageing. Begin by eliminating processed foods and added sugar from your diet, focusing instead on whole, nutrient-dense options such as fruits, vegetables, whole grains and lean proteins.

Quitting sugar can be tough. To help break the cycle of sugar addiction, including mental addiction, consider reading Allen Carr's book *The Easy Way to Quit Sugar*.

You don't need to overhaul your diet –
simply shorten your eating window to eight
hours a day to start reaping the benefits.

TIME YOUR MEALS

When you eat may be just as important as what you eat. Intermittent fasting (also known as time-restricted eating) is a simple strategy that involves eating within a set window of time each day – giving your body regular breaks from digestion to focus on repair. Studies show it can support metabolic health, reduce inflammation and induce autophagy – the cellular 'spring cleaning' that helps remove damaged cells and promote longevity. One popular intermittent fasting method is the 16:8 approach, where you limit your intake of foods to a set window of eight hours per day. You then abstain from food for the remaining sixteen hours (drinking water, black coffee or tea during the fast is fine). Another approach is the 5:2 method, where you eat as normal for five days a week, then reduce calorie intake to 500–800 calories on two non-consecutive days.

However, intermittent fasting isn't for everyone, particularly women with hormone imbalances, low energy or a history of disordered eating. Women's bodies are more sensitive to perceived energy deficits, especially during perimenopause or reproductive years, which can affect cortisol, thyroid and reproductive hormone balance. For some, fasting can throw off cortisol levels, slow down thyroid function or interfere with ovulation and cycle regularity.

That said, it's normal to feel a little off the first time you try it. Around twelve to sixteen hours into a fast, your body starts switching from burning glucose to burning fat. This process produces ketones, which your brain can use for fuel. That's why many people actually feel more focused and energized during a fast. With proper support, extended fasts have even shown promising results for things like insulin resistance, cellular repair and certain cancer therapies. Fasting can also support your mitochondria, the energy centres of your cells. It helps clean out damaged ones (a process called mitophagy) and encourages the growth of new, healthier mitochondria. This can mean better energy, less inflammation and stronger long-term health.

Regardless of whether you choose to fast or not, it's best to avoid late-night eating. Eating close to bedtime can interfere with your body's natural circadian rhythms and impact the quality of your sleep.

SIP SMART

Hydration is one of the simplest, yet most overlooked, ways to support your health every day. Water helps regulate body temperature, keep digestion running smoothly and transport nutrients where they're needed. Drinking enough water each day can also help with weight management by helping you differentiate between hunger and thirst. Dehydration, on the other hand, can lead to fatigue, headaches, poor concentration and impaired cognitive function. Additionally, chronic dehydration is associated with an increased risk of kidney disease and urinary tract infections, particularly in older adults.

Modern water is often heavily filtered and stripped of minerals like magnesium and potassium electrolytes that help regulate hydration at the cellular level. While plain water can still hydrate you, the absence of these minerals may reduce how efficiently your body absorbs and retains it, especially in situations of stress, exertion or mineral deficiency. Over time, this may contribute to subtle, chronic dehydration.

You may not feel thirsty, but low-grade dehydration is incredibly common. It can show up as headaches, fatigue, brain fog, dry skin, low mood and even sluggish digestion. Most people walk around mildly dehydrated every day without realizing it.

Here's how to hydrate more effectively:

- Add minerals to your water. A pinch of Celtic Sea Salt in your glass helps water enter your cells more efficiently. It contains magnesium, potassium and over seventy trace minerals that support hydration, energy and the nervous system.

- Start your day with water. Aim for 500–750 ml within thirty minutes of waking up to replenish your body system after sleep and kickstart cellular hydration.

- Try hydrogen water. Some early studies suggest that hydrogen-infused water – made using tablets or a hydrogen-generating bottle – may support cellular repair and reduce oxidative stress.

DITCH THE DRINK

Some people may defend alcohol for its alleged health benefits, citing studies that have linked moderate alcohol consumption with lower risk of heart disease. Some may also consider red wine 'healthy' because it contains the antioxidant resveratrol, which studies show could extend lifespan.

However, a study published in the *Lancet* has shown that no amount of alcohol is safe. Even a low intake increases the risk of cancer, liver damage and cognitive decline. Moreover, alcohol is a depressant that can disrupt brain chemistry, worsen mental health and raise blood sugar. It's also one of the leading risk factors for disease and premature death worldwide.

Yes, red wine contains resveratrol – but only in small amounts, typically less than 2 mg per glass. Most studies suggesting health benefits use doses of 100–500 mg or more – levels that would require drinking 50–250 glasses per day. For any meaningful effect, supplementation is likely a more practical option.

SAVOUR WITHOUT SACRIFICE

It is wise to replace some (or all!) of your alcoholic beverages with healthier, more nourishing alternatives – such as sparkling water, herbal teas or kombucha. These options can help satisfy the need for a social or sensory ritual without the downsides of alcohol. In fact, creating a new set of 'go-to' drinks can help you feel just as included in social situations – without the sluggishness, regret or health risks that alcohol can bring.

In social settings, planning ahead is key. Decide in advance what you will drink and stick to your plan. More and more venues now offer sophisticated alcohol-free mocktails and wines, as well as botanical spirits that feel festive without the hangover. Bringing your own favourite alcohol-free option to parties can also help remove any pressure or temptation.

Remind yourself that eliminating alcohol does not mean you're missing out – on the contrary, it can enhance your health, relationships and personal growth. If you rely on alcohol to cope with stress or social anxiety, consider healthier coping strategies or seek professional support. However, if you are not ready to wave goodbye to alcohol, consider limiting your intake to one or two glasses of red wine per week.

BE SMART WITH CAFFEINE

Many people rely on their daily cup (or three) of caffeine for focus, mood and energy. Caffeine is linked with increased alertness, enhanced concentration and even reduced risk of conditions like Parkinson's disease. Some research even suggests that moderate caffeine consumption may support long-term health and longevity. But as with most things, context and dose matter.

Too much caffeine may reduce brain plasticity (the brain's ability to form new connections, especially in response to learning). It can also lead to diminished cognitive function, increased stress hormone levels and negatively impact the quality of sleep.

Finally, caffeine can be habit-forming, which is why people feel compelled to consume it daily to avoid energy slumps and maintain alertness throughout the day – otherwise, withdrawal symptoms such as headaches, fatigue and irritability can kick in. There's a genetic component to this: people who carry certain variants of the CYP1A2 gene may metabolize caffeine more slowly.

This means a single espresso or black tea could leave you feeling jittery, anxious or wide awake at night, while someone else processes it without issue. So instead of quitting cold turkey, consider being more mindful of caffeine.

Try reducing your intake or avoiding caffeine after 2 p.m. (the half-life of caffeine is about five to six hours). And if you're curious, testing for CPY1A2 variants can offer insight into how your body handles it.

SUPERCHARGE YOUR DIET WITH SUPPLEMENTS

You've now learned how to eat for longevity and how to personalize your nutrition to fit your body's needs. But even the most nutrient-dense diet isn't always enough. Modern agriculture has led to soil depletion. Chronic stress and certain medications can impair nutrient absorption. And sometimes, our stage of life or genetic makeup increases our demand for specific vitamins or minerals.

This is where supplements can play a strategic role. While supplements alone won't transform your health, they are a powerful tool for filling any gaps in an already balanced diet and lifestyle. On the next pages you will find the top five supplements for general wellbeing, as well as the top seven supplements for longevity.

GENERAL HEALTH SUPPLEMENTS

METHYLATED B-VITAMINS

B-vitamins are essential for DNA repair, energy metabolism and cellular function. They also support brain health, potentially reducing the risk of anxiety and depression, as well as cognitive decline. Finally, B-vitamins play an important role in energy metabolism and may help reduce fatigue. Some individuals with genetic variants that affect methylation may benefit from additional nutritional support, such as methylated B-vitamins, since their bodies may struggle to convert standard forms into their active, usable forms.

Methylated B-vitamins bypass the need for this conversion and are therefore easier to absorb and utilize. Even if you don't have the MTHFR gene mutation, you can still benefit from the active methylated forms of B-vitamins, as they're more readily absorbed and used by the body. For ease of consumption look for B-vitamins which are sold as a vitamin complex, so you don't have to purchase each vitamin individually.

Suggested adult dosages:

- Vitamin B2: 1.3 mg per day.

- Vitamin B6: 1.3 mg per day.

- Vitamin B9: 400 mcg (micrograms) per day.

- Vitamin B12: 2.4 mcg (micrograms) per day.

VITAMIN D

Vitamin D is often called the 'sunshine vitamin' – but it's also a powerful hormone. Yet nearly 40 per cent of Europeans (and a large number of people globally, especially those who live in northern latitudes or spend most of their time indoors) are deficient in vitamin D. This vitamin is essential for maintaining strong bones, supporting immune function and regulating mood. It also enhances the pathogen-fighting effects of white blood cells that are crucial in the body's defence against infections. Low levels of vitamin D are associated with mood disorders, including depression and seasonal affective disorder (SAD).

Because it's difficult to get enough vitamin D from food alone, and sun exposure isn't always possible, supplementation is often recommended. The suggested adult dosage is 5,000 IU (International Unit) per day, especially for those with limited sun exposure.

MAGNESIUM

Some studies suggest around 70 per cent of the UK population have low magnesium levels, and that number may be even higher among those with chronic stress or high physical demands. Magnesium is involved in over 300 enzymatic reactions, including those that regulate energy production, muscle and nerve function, sleep and mood. It is also required to activate vitamin D. Low magnesium levels are linked to poor sleep, heightened stress response, muscle cramps and even insulin resistance. Many people find that increasing magnesium levels improves their sleep quality, reduces anxiety and helps them wind down more easily at night.

There are several forms of magnesium, each with slightly different effects:

- Magnesium glycinate: gentle on the gut, calming, great for stress and sleep.

- Magnesium citrate: supports digestive regularity.

- Magnesium threonate: may support cognitive health and brain function.

Suggested adult dosage of *elemental* magnesium: 400 mg per day

ALPHA LIPOIC ACID (ALA)

Alpha lipoic acid (ALA) is a potent antioxidant that helps protect the body by neutralizing free radicals – unstable molecules that are naturally produced during metabolism and can damage cells, proteins and DNA if left unchecked. It helps regenerate other antioxidants like vitamins C and E. In addition, ALA may help improve insulin sensitivity, reduce the risk of neurodegenerative conditions such as Parkinson's disease and boost energy production at the cellular level.

Suggested adult dosage: 600 mg per day

RHODIOLA ROSEA

Rhodiola rosea is an adaptogenic herb native to the mountainous regions of Europe and Asia. It has been used for centuries to support mental resilience, stamina and mood – especially in high-stress environments. Rhodiola rosea extends lifespan in animal research for reasons that scientists have not completely understood yet. Studies in humans show that it can help improve learning and memory function, as well as reduce fatigue, making it ideal for students and people with demanding jobs. Start with a lower dose (200 mg, for example) to assess tolerance before increasing if needed. It is best taken early in the day to avoid potential interference with sleep.

Suggested adult dosage: 200–600 mg per day

LONGEVITY SUPPLEMENTS

NMN (NICOTINAMIDE MONONUCLEOTIDE)

NMN helps increase levels of NAD+ (nicotinamide adenine dinucleotide), a molecule critical for energy production, DNA repair and healthy cellular function. NAD+ levels decline significantly with age, and this decline has been linked with fatigue, reduced metabolic function and increased risk of chronic disease. Because NAD+ is too large to enter our cells directly, supplementing with precursors like NMN has become a promising workaround. NMN is more easily absorbed and can be converted to NAD+ inside cells. Most of the research on NMN comes from animal studies, yet human trials are emerging and suggest that NMN may support metabolic health and improve markers like muscle strength, aerobic capacity and insulin sensitivity. There's also some evidence that NMN may help support healthy gut microbiota and enhance DNA repair, two factors linked to healthy ageing.

Suggested adult dosage: 1 g per day (take together with resveratrol, as they work in synergy)

RESVERATROL

Resveratrol is a powerful antioxidant found in red grapes, berries and peanuts, known for its anti-inflammatory properties. It's been studied for its potential to support heart health, improve insulin sensitivity and activate sirtuins – proteins linked to cellular repair and longevity. It also helps improve energy metabolism and enhance resistance to stress. In animals, resveratrol has shown promise in slowing ageing and even suppressing cancer cell growth. Resveratrol is poorly absorbed, and high doses are not easily achieved through food, so supplementation is recommended.

Suggested adult dosage: 1 g per day (take together with NMN, as they work in synergy)

HYALURONIC ACID

Hyaluronic acid is a naturally occurring molecule found in our skin and joints, best known for its ability to hold up to 1,000 times its weight in water. It helps keep our skin hydrated, smooth and plump – essentially acting like a moisture magnet. As we age, hyaluronic acid levels decline, which contributes to dryness, fine lines and joint stiffness.

Research has shown that oral ingestion of hyaluronic acid for twelve weeks may improve skin hydration and elasticity, as well as the appearance of wrinkles. Studies also show that hyaluronic acid can improve the symptoms of osteoarthritis and associated structural damage.

Suggested adult dosage: 120 mg per day

FISETIN

Fisetin is a plant compound found in vegetables and fruits, and most abundantly in apples and strawberries. It's classified as a senolytic, meaning it helps the body clear out senescent cells: old, dysfunctional cells that no longer divide but refuse to die. These cells cause trouble by releasing inflammatory molecules that not only damage nearby tissues but can trigger healthy neighbouring cells to become senescent too – a dangerous biological 'bystander effect'.

Over time, as immune function declines, these cells accumulate and contribute to ageing and chronic disease. Fisetin may help reduce this cellular burden, making it easier for the immune system to stay in control. Animal studies show it may reduce inflammation, support brain health and extend lifespan. Human clinical research is underway.

Suggested adult dosage: 100 mg per day

SPERMIDINE

Spermidine is a naturally occurring compound found in foods such as soybeans, mushrooms and aged cheese. Spermidine helps trigger autophagy, the body's natural process for clearing out old, damaged cells. This may support heart health, brain function and lifespan. Studies have also shown that spermidine can help alleviate obesity and other diseases in both animals and humans.

Suggested adult dosage: 5 mg per day

COQ10

Coenzyme Q10 is vital for energy production in your mitochondria, your cells' power plants. Levels naturally decline with age and may be depleted by statins or chronic stress. CoQ10 supports cardiovascular health, fertility and athletic performance.

Suggested daily dosage: 100–200 mg of *ubiquinol* (the active form of CoQ10)

GLUTATHIONE

Often called the body's 'master antioxidant', glutathione plays a central role in detoxification, immune resilience and mitochondrial function. It helps neutralize toxins and supports liver health, especially during times of oxidative stress or chronic exposure.

Look for liposomal glutathione for better absorption, or consider NAC (N-acetylcysteine), a precursor that helps your body produce its own.

Suggested daily dosage:

- Glutathione: 250–500 mg
- NAC (as an alternative): 600–1,200 mg

The best supplement routine is one that fits your body, lifestyle and personal requirements. Start with lab work to identify any deficiencies and work with a trusted practitioner (whether a doctor, dietitian or functional provider) to guide your choices. Always check for interactions if you're on medication, and choose high-quality, well-absorbed supplement forms. Remember, supplements are meant to support your system, not replace the foundations of health like food, movement, sleep and stress management.

CHAPTER SUMMARY

What you eat, and how you eat it, has a profound impact on how you age. This chapter explored the science of nutrient density, blood sugar regulation, inflammation and cellular health, with a focus on personalization over perfection. It's not about following strict diets or cutting out entire food groups but about tuning in to how your body responds to different foods, and making informed choices that support your energy, health and longevity. From supporting your methylation pathways and feeding your mitochondria to upgrading hydration and ditching processed foods, each shift you make is a signal to your body: healing can begin. Quality matters. Timing matters. Your biology is always listening, and food is one of your most powerful levers.

QUICK RECAP: EAT FOR LONGEVITY

- Prioritize whole, nutrient-dense foods.

- Focus on glucose balance – use food pairing, movement and protein-first meals.

- Support methylation with dark leafy greens, beetroot and methylated B-vitamins.

- Upgrade hydration: add Celtic Sea Salt or minerals and try hydrogen water for extra support.

- Use targeted supplements (like magnesium, omega-3, vitamin D, CoQ10 and glutathione) to support energy, detox and repair.

- Explore intermittent fasting to activate autophagy and give your body time to reset.

'Muscle is your metabolic currency. The more you have, the better you age.'

Dr Gabrielle Lyon

Author of the bestselling book
Forever Strong

MOVE

If you want to stay younger for longer, build muscle. Muscle is far more than just tissue that helps you move – it's a metabolically active organ that plays a central role in ageing well. It's the largest site of glucose disposal in your body and helps stabilize blood sugar, prevent insulin resistance and regulate energy and mood.

It produces anti-inflammatory molecules called myokines, which protect your brain, strengthen your immune system and help you recover faster from stress, injury and illness. It's the only thing that can stop, slow or even reverse sarcopenia – the age-related loss of muscle that begins in your thirties, accelerates in your forties and fifties, and drastically impacts your healthspan if left unaddressed.

Research shows that simply maintaining more muscle as you age is associated with a lower risk of chronic disease, improved brain function and a longer lifespan. In fact, low muscle mass is now considered a greater predictor of early death than obesity or smoking in older adults. Put simply: muscle is the organ of longevity. It protects you from nearly every major disease of ageing – including type 2 diabetes, heart disease, osteoporosis, cognitive decline – and can even activate genes involved in metabolism and cellular repair.

Regular strength-building exercise also improves your sleep. By promoting deeper, restorative slow-wave sleep, it helps your body balance hormones overnight, clear excess glucose from your blood and support brain detox through the glymphatic system – a recently discovered network that acts as the brain's night-time cleaning crew. However, keep in mind that strenuous workouts within four hours of bedtime may impair sleep quality. Opt for lighter movement in the evening or finish earlier in the day for more restful nights.

While all movement has value, not all movement builds muscle. The single most powerful thing you can do for your future self is to build and preserve muscle – especially after forty, when the risk of sarcopenia and metabolic decline increases dramatically. Pilates, yoga and gentle movement are powerful tools for flexibility, recovery and nervous system balance – but they aren't substitutes for focused, progressive resistance training that challenges your muscle tissue.

Longevity isn't driven by discipline; it's built on what you enjoy enough to keep doing. Think back to what you loved as a kid. Was it running, riding a bike, climbing or dancing? The more you enjoy your training, the more likely you are to keep going – and consistency is what changes everything. A balanced mix of strength training, restorative movement and joyful physical activity can recalibrate your metabolism, protect your brain and build the energy and resilience you need to chase your grandkids, sleep well, recover quickly and stay mentally sharp well into your later years.

MUSCLE IS YOUR LONGEVITY CURRENCY

So what does 'strength training' entail? It doesn't mean maxing out on day one – it means training at a level that challenges your muscles enough to stimulate growth. One useful benchmark is your rep max: the number of reps you can perform with good form before reaching fatigue. You'll know you have found the right weight to train with when you can do eight to twelve reps, and the final two reps feel hard but doable, without breaking form. That's your personal sweet spot. Over time, increase the load or volume (reps) to continue progressing and building muscle mass.

Your muscle is your body's largest metabolic organ – essential for glucose control, mitochondrial health and insulin sensitivity. This is because skeletal muscle acts as a major storage site for glucose, pulling sugar out of the bloodstream and storing it as glycogen. The more muscle you have, and the more you use it, the more efficiently you can clear blood sugar after your meals. It also protects your brain through the release of myokines, increases bone density, regulates blood sugar and resists disease. It also supports cognitive clarity, immune function and recovery from physical or emotional stress. Muscle doesn't only keep you upright, it keeps you thinking clearly and moving with power. Aim for at least two full-body resistance sessions per week – enough to stimulate adaptation, maintain muscle mass and support healthy ageing.

So how can you check your progress? Experts like Dr Gabrielle Lyon and Dr Peter Attia recommend maintaining enough strength to deadlift your bodyweight, carry groceries upstairs or get up from the floor without assistance – not because it's impressive but because it's protective. Another simple, science-backed indicator of healthy ageing? Grip strength.

Grip strength, or the ability of your hand and forearm to exert force when grasping or holding an object, correlates with total body muscle mass, heart health and even cognitive function. In fact, studies have shown that low grip strength is linked to higher risk of all-cause mortality, frailty and earlier onset of disease. It's considered by many researchers to be a reliable 'biomarker of ageing' as a better grip strength is linked with a slower pace of biological ageing.

Grip strength is easy to test with a handheld dynamometer, but even tracking how easily you can open jars, carry heavy bags or hang from a bar can give you a feel for where you stand. If you want to improve your grip strength, prioritize exercises like dead hangs, farmer's carries, kettlebell work and pull movements like rows or chin-ups.

If weights feel intimidating, start with resistance bands or your own bodyweight. The method matters less than the message your body receives by training for strength – and eating to keep it. Make sure you're pairing your strength training with meals rich in protein, so your body has the raw materials to repair, grow and stay metabolically sharp.

CARDIO

While strength training builds your metabolic engine, aerobic activity keeps it running. Cardio-based movement like brisk walking, cycling, swimming, running or dancing strengthens your heart, lungs and vascular system. It's also one of the most well-researched tools for preventing heart disease and supporting brain health as you age. Regular aerobic exercise improves blood flow and oxygen delivery to the brain, which supports memory, executive function and the growth of new neurons – especially in areas affected by ageing, like the hippocampus. Studies show it can reduce the risk of cognitive decline and dementia, especially when done consistently over time.

For added benefit in less time, you can experiment with high-intensity interval training (HIIT): short bursts of exertion followed by rest or low effort. A simple protocol might include cycling or sprinting for thirty seconds, then recovering for fifteen to thirty seconds and repeated for ten to fifteen minutes.

HIIT improves endurance capacity, supports fat loss while preserving muscle mass and stimulates the release of brain-derived neurotrophic factor (BDNF), a key molecule in neuroplasticity and cognitive function.

TAKE A WALK

Once strength is part of your weekly routine, walking becomes additional support for your brain, blood sugar, nervous system and breath. Just five to ten minutes of walking after meals can reduce glucose spikes and encourage hormone balance. Walking is also great for cardiovascular health and reducing mortality risk. However, it does very little to preserve or build muscle mass – which is why strength training remains essential. You don't necessarily need 10,000 steps a day – that number came from a Japanese 1960s ad campaign, not from scientific evidence. Research shows benefits begin at around 2,500 steps and tend to plateau between 6,000 and 8,000 steps, especially as we age.

Walking isn't just a physical act, it's a reset for your nervous system too. Rhythmic movement helps regulate stress, support vagal tone and shift you out of fight-or-flight into a calmer state. Research has also linked walking with improved mental clarity and creativity. The average increase in creative ideas was around 60 per cent in people who walked compared to their sedentary counterparts. For example, Steve Jobs and Mark Zuckerberg were often seen holding walking meetings.

Want to amplify the benefits even more? Walk in nature. Trees release phytoncides – bioactive compounds that serve as a natural defence system against bacteria, fungi and insects. When humans inhale these compounds, especially in biodiverse forests, they have a measurable effect on our physiology. Phytoncides increase natural killer (NK) cell activity, which strengthens immune defences against viruses and abnormal cells. They also help lower cortisol levels, support nervous system regulation and promote parasympathetic dominance – your rest-and-digest state – by reducing heart rate and blood pressure and improving heart rate variability (HRV). Over time, this nervous system recalibration may even enhance sleep quality by supporting melatonin-related pathways.

It's no wonder forest air has been shown to reduce anxiety, improve mood and leave people feeling both grounded and energized. And when you walk with someone you love, the benefits compound – strong relationships are the single most powerful predictor of long-term health and happiness. In the end, it's not about hitting a specific number. It's about rhythm, restoration and remembering that movement can be both healing and incredibly simple.

DAILY MOVEMENT IN REAL LIFE

Everyday life offers countless chances to nourish your body through motion. If you enjoy tracking your physical activity, most smartphones and wearable devices will estimate your step count. On average, 10,000 steps equal about ninety minutes of walking, but even half that can offer significant health benefits. Most people log 3,500–5,000 steps just through errands, dog-walking, chores, or commuting – so you may be closer to the goal than you think.

Looking to add more movement into your day? Go for short walks after meals. Purchase a walking pad. Always take the stairs. Try wall push-ups, air squats or walking lunges between meetings or while waiting for dinner to cook. These short bursts of movement help build muscle and improve glucose uptake.

Frequent movement also acts as a hormetic stressor – a beneficial form of stress that nudges your body to boost mitochondrial function and build metabolic flexibility. When spaced throughout the day, these micro-movements send a powerful biological signal: adapt, repair and grow stronger.

DIVERSIFY YOUR EXERCISE

While strength training is the cornerstone of healthy ageing, other forms of movement play essential supporting roles. Aerobic exercise keeps your heart and lungs strong, supports circulation and delivers oxygen to your brain. Practices like mobility work, mind–body movement and stretching help maintain joint health, flexibility and coordination. While they won't replace the need for progressive resistance training, they offer powerful benefits for nervous system regulation, posture and injury prevention when practised consistently.

The more ways you move, the more resilient your body becomes. Each type of movement activates different systems – from your heart to your lymph, to your brain. Explore what feels good and let your routine evolve with the seasons of your life.

HOW MUCH SHOULD YOU EXERCISE?

Exercise offers one of the highest returns on investment in all of health. Just a few hours a week can buy you years of independence, sharper thinking and more time doing what you love. But too little and your body starts to weaken; too much, and you risk burnout or injury. Engaging in the right amount of physical activity is key to reaping long-term benefits. Yet the hard truth is most people aren't moving enough. A 2022 WHO report found that more than 1 in 4 adults worldwide fail to meet the minimum physical activity guidelines. Sedentary behaviour – especially prolonged sitting – has become the norm.

But what is the right amount of exercise? The consensus is at least 150 minutes of moderate-intensity activity per week, which is about twenty minutes per day. Make at least two of those sessions strength training to maintain muscle mass. From there, you can add one or two HIIT sessions per week – they can be as short as seven minutes and can take place at the end of your usual workouts. A dedicated mobility or stretching session, even a single session each week, is enough to make a difference.

However, the best plan is the one you actually follow. When it comes to longevity, consistency trumps perfection. You don't need to run marathons, but you need to move regularly if you want to carry your groceries with ease at seventy-five, climb stairs confidently at eighty or chase your grandkids through the garden without joint pain.

But what if you don't have the energy to start? That's not a failure of willpower – it could be a signal from your mitochondria. These tiny powerhouses inside your cells fuel everything from movement and memory to hormone production and repair. When mitochondria are underfed, overworked or inflamed, your body feels it: exhaustion, brain fog, poor sleep or simply not feeling like yourself anymore. Food, stress, toxins and even the information you consume, all shape how well your mitochondria function.

If this resonates, start with nourishment. Replenish your body with nutrient-dense foods, targeted supplements (based on testing) and nervous system support. Let walking be your entry point. Just ten to fifteen minutes a day can gently awaken your energy system without overloading it.

Because once energy begins to return, even just a little, momentum builds. Within a few weeks of consistent, gentle movement, you may notice better sleep, sharper focus and a more stable mood. Within a month, friends may comment on your radiant energy. By three months, your posture, stamina and clarity will speak for themselves. You'll get to resistance training and HIIT when your body is ready – but first, build the foundation: healthy, resilient mitochondria. That journey starts now.

Remember, exercise doesn't have to be hard or painful to be effective. Physical activity at an exertion level of 60–80 per cent of your maximum capacity (meaning you can still have a light conversation) is enough to notice benefits. When you are ready, you can add in one or two HIIT sessions per week – where your maximum exertion reaches up to 90–95 per cent of your maximum capacity.

Consistency, not intensity, is key, so try to find something that you enjoy and can fit into your lifestyle – then keep at it! Regularly engaging even in small amounts of exercise can provide significant health benefits over time.

MIND-BODY PRACTICES

Movement isn't just physical. It's also neurological and emotional. Alongside your physical training, mind–body practices help upgrade something that many longevity plans overlook: your nervous system. A growing number of studies show that mind–body practices improve brain neuroplasticity, influence gene expression at the cellular level and help regulate stress-related pathways. The latter can help us feel calmer by reducing physical symptoms of stress (such as increased heart rate, muscle tension and rapid breathing) and balancing levels of 'stress' hormones such as cortisol.

This is where real resilience is built, not just in your muscles or HRV, but in how you respond to life. Breathwork, meditation, yoga and Qigong aren't gentle add-ons. They're performance tools that restore your calm, sharpen focus and reset the physiological stress response that ages your body from the inside out. Unlike your other workouts, the goal here isn't muscle growth or calorie burn, it's to create coherence – where breath, movement and intention work in sync to shift the brain and body into a state of safety and restoration.

YOGA

At its best, yoga isn't a workout – it's a reset. A moving meditation that builds strength, flexibility and awareness all at once. And it does more than lengthen your hamstrings. Studies show that yoga can positively influence both the body and the mind. For example, it can relieve chronic pain in the lower back and neck, as well as symptoms of arthritis.

Yoga can also literally change your brain chemistry for the better. Regular yoga increases activity in the parts of the brain (anterior cingulate cortex and the medial prefrontal cortex) that are associated with empathy, gratitude and emotional regulation. You may walk into a session with a racing mind and walk out grounded, clear and emotionally lighter.

To notice improvements in flexibility, strength and mental clarity, aim to incorporate yoga in short daily sessions of ten to twenty minutes about five to six times a week. Alternatively, do longer sessions of sixty to ninety minutes two to three times a week.

QIGONG

Qigong is a powerful Chinese health practice that is thousands of years old and aligns breath, movement and awareness to promote both vitality and healing. Through fluid, intentional movements and rhythmic breathing, Qigong taps into your body's energy grid – what ancient medicine calls *qi* (the vital life force), and which, according to traditional Chinese medicine, flows through the human body and all living things.

It is gentle enough to do daily and potent enough to reduce chronic pain, improve immune markers and lift symptoms of anxiety and depression. That's the power of somatic rhythm – where the body leads, the mind follows.

Practising Qigong three to five times a week provides health benefits, but daily practice, even for just ten to twenty minutes, generally offers the most noticeable improvements in relaxation and wellbeing.

You don't need to choose one modality or get it perfect. Try different forms. See how your body responds. A few minutes a day of breath-led movement, of deep nervous system reset, can radically shift how you experience your life, your energy and your longevity. Because the reality is: you can eat every superfood and take every supplement, but if your body is stuck in a stress loop, it will never feel safe enough to activate its fullest healing potential.

HORMETIC HEAT AND COLD: TRAIN YOUR BODY'S ADAPTATION SYSTEMS

Hot and cold therapies have gained popularity for their ability to enhance resilience and cellular function. When used strategically, temperature extremes act as controlled stressors that stimulate mitochondrial health, reduce inflammation and support detoxification – especially via the liver, which plays a central role in hormonal balance, gut health and waste elimination. And in a world wrought with environmental toxins, processed food and endocrine disruptors, your detox systems need all the support they can get.

THE POWER OF SWEAT

There's something deeply restorative about heat. Whether it's through sauna, infrared or steam – thermal therapy nudges your body to release stress, improve circulation and activate cellular pathways tied to resilience and repair.

Heat works by gently raising your core temperature, increasing circulation and activating your mitochondria. Gently raising your core temperature supports mitochondrial function and triggers sweating – a process that helps eliminate trace toxins and reduce fluid retention. While your liver does the heavy lifting of detoxification, sweating can provide supportive relief, especially when you're feeling bloated, fatigued, foggy or hormonally out of balance. When your detox pathways are sluggish, regular heat exposure can help reset the system.

Sauna also activates heat shock proteins, cellular guardians that protect your body from damage and support longevity. In fact, regular sauna use has been linked to reduced risk of dementia, better heart health and lower all-cause mortality in multiple large-scale studies.

THE CASE FOR COLD
(WITH CAVEATS)

If heat is a gentle exhale, cold is a sharp inhale. It pulls you into the present, clears your mind and resets your nervous system almost instantly. Just a few minutes of cold exposure, whether through a plunge, a cold shower or cryotherapy, can increase dopamine, lower inflammation and improve mitochondrial function. Cold also activates brown fat, a metabolically active tissue that burns calories to generate heat. This supports blood sugar regulation, metabolic flexibility and even fat loss. Many people report better energy, focus and mood with regular exposure.

Cold exposure may also improve mental health because it causes an increase in norepinephrine and dopamine, neurotransmitters associated with enhanced mood. But it's not without nuance, especially for women. Due to hormonal cycles and naturally higher parasympathetic tone, women may be more sensitive to the stress load of cold exposure. For those in their reproductive years or with thyroid or adrenal concerns, too much cold can disrupt rather than support hormonal balance. It's best used sparingly, intentionally and always according to how your body feels that day.

For those who want to try cold therapy, start with contrast showers: brief blasts of cold after a hot shower can improve circulation, boost alertness and support vascular flexibility. If you're experimenting with plunges, keep them short (up to ten minutes) and infrequent (two or three times per week). Cryotherapy is another option for those looking for inflammation or pain relief without full water immersion, but it's expensive and often less accessible.

HOT AND COLD THERAPY: SAFETY TIPS AND GUIDELINES

Heat and cold therapies can be powerful tools for nervous system regulation, detoxification and cellular health. Think of them as tuning forks for your body. They can help you shift between stress and relaxation, activation and recovery. Always start slow, prioritize safety and consult your doctor if you have a heart condition. For most people, short, consistent sessions beat long, extreme ones.

CHAPTER SUMMARY

Muscle is your organ of longevity. It's a powerful metabolic reserve that protects you as you age. Maintaining lean muscle helps regulate blood sugar, reduce inflammation, support hormone balance and even lower your risk of chronic disease. Strength training is one of the most protective habits you can build, especially as you enter midlife and beyond. Aim for two or more sessions each week that challenge your muscles through resistance, whether with weights, bands or your own body weight.

Once strength is part of your weekly routine, small amounts of daily movement like walking can amplify the benefits. A short fifteen- to twenty-five-minute walk improves glucose control, boosts cardiovascular health and enhances brain function. Even better: a quick walk after meals can reduce blood sugar spikes and support digestive flow. While the popular 10,000-step goal is arbitrary, research shows the real benefits begin around 2,500 steps and tend to plateau near 7,500 steps.

Round out your movement with practices that support recovery and nervous system health. Yoga, Qigong and other mind–body approaches can improve mobility, reduce stress and bring a sense of calm. Heat therapy – like sauna use – can support detoxification, while also aiding stress recovery. It can be a helpful complement for those experiencing sluggish energy, skin issues or hormone fluctuations. Cold therapy may support mitochondrial health and mood regulation, but it needs to be used strategically, particularly for women navigating hormonal balance. Always listen to your body.

In the end, movement is about building a body that works for you. One that's strong, steady and resilient for decades to come.

'Sleep is the single most effective thing we can do to reset our brain and body health each day.'

Dr Matthew Walker

Author of the bestselling book *Why We Sleep*

SLEEP

It's 10.47 p.m. You're tired but still scrolling. The glow of your phone floods your face as you skim emails or social media. Minutes blur into an hour. When the alarm blares six hours later, you feel groggy, wired but tired ... and you reach for your phone again. Worse than simply being a habit, this is a circadian disruption. Blue light from screens suppresses melatonin, the hormone that signals your body to wind down. Without that signal, your internal clock – the circadian rhythm – falls out of sync. Sleep onset is delayed. Hormones stay dysregulated. Your mitochondria miss their repair window. Sleep isn't just rest, it's a nightly system reset. Poor sleep compromises glucose regulation, raises inflammation, lowers HRV and impairs detoxification. Even one night of insufficient sleep can spike cortisol and disrupt insulin sensitivity.

The good news? Your body is wired for rhythm. This chapter will offer practical strategies to rebuild the foundation of long-term energy, focus and lasting health.

WHY SLEEP IS THE ULTIMATE LONGEVITY TOOL

Sleep is one of the most powerful, accessible tools you have to extend your healthspan. Every night, the body shifts into a phase of intensive biological repair. Mitochondria, the powerhouses of our cells, use this time to recover from oxidative stress and restore energy capacity. Key hormones cycle and recalibrate: melatonin rises to anchor circadian rhythm and provide antioxidant defence, growth hormone surges to stimulate tissue repair and cortisol is reset to prepare the body for morning alertness. The liver increases detoxification activity, processing the metabolic waste accumulated during the day. Meanwhile, the brain enters a unique state where it cleans itself through the glymphatic system, flushing out neurotoxins like beta-amyloid, and rebalancing neurotransmitters such as dopamine and serotonin.

Sleep also plays a central role in regulating glucose metabolism. During deep sleep, insulin sensitivity improves, glucose uptake is optimized and blood sugar levels stabilize — helping to prevent the spikes and crashes that drive inflammation, weight gain and hormonal imbalance.

Poor sleep disrupts this entire sequence, leading to mitochondrial dysfunction, reduced HRV, impaired immune response and elevated inflammation markers like CRP. Studies have shown that adults need at least seven to nine hours of sleep each night. Even a single night of insufficient sleep can lower natural killer cells, a type of immune cell that helps detect and destroy abnormal cells, by up to 70 per cent. Research shows people who don't get enough sleep are up to four times more likely to get sick after being exposed to a virus. Over time, the wear and tear add up. Your body starts ageing faster, even if everything looks fine on the outside.

The link between sleep and heart health is striking. One study found that when daylight saving time 'springs forward', resulting in an hour of lost sleep, heart attacks jump up by 24 per cent the very next day. When an hour of sleep is gained in autumn, heart attacks drop by 21 per cent.

At the centre of this system is your circadian rhythm: the body's internal twenty-four-hour clock, which governs sleep, hormone release, metabolism, body temperature and more. When sleep is aligned with your circadian rhythm, all systems synchronize for maximum recovery and resilience. But when sleep is irregular, delayed or insufficient, the entire biological orchestra falls out of tune.

If you want to support your mitochondria, balance your hormones, sharpen your cognition, lower your biological age and protect your long-term vitality – it starts with sleep. It's so much more than just rest. It's repair, detox, regulation and rejuvenation. It's the foundation for everything else.

DO OLDER ADULTS NEED LESS SLEEP?

Not exactly, but it can feel that way. What happens is this: as you age, your body has a harder time getting the kind of sleep it needs. The ability to reach deep, restorative sleep often fades with age, and the total amount of sleep may become lighter and more broken up.

This change can begin as early as midlife. As we get older, shifts in hormones, reduced oxygen levels and changes in methylation can all affect sleep depth and quality. Deep sleep tends to get shorter, and the brain doesn't recover as well overnight. That can lead to lower levels of melatonin, testosterone and growth hormone – three hormones that naturally decline with age and are essential for energy, strength and resilience. There's growing research suggesting that poor sleep might not just be a symptom of ageing, it may actually make the ageing process faster.

Your genes can also play a role. Some people have DNA variations that make them more prone to anxiety, poor melatonin production or disrupted sleep cycles. For example, variations in the MTHFR gene may be linked to higher rates of sleep trouble. But this doesn't mean poor sleep is inevitable. You can learn more about your body by testing for your sleep chronotype or genetic markers related to sleep, which can help you find better strategies for recovery.

If falling or staying asleep is a challenge, adding 5-HTP may help. This supplement can increase serotonin, which supports melatonin production and may improve sleep quality. Still, sleep issues are rarely caused by just one thing. Blood sugar swings, stress, light exposure at night and irregular habits often have a bigger impact than genes alone.

Instead of viewing poor sleep as an expected part of ageing, treat it as something you can work on. Improving sleep now will help protect your memory, mood and physical health for years to come.

THE ANATOMY OF SLEEP

Sleep unfolds in structured, repeating ninety-minute cycles, each with distinct biological roles. These cycles include three non-REM stages (N1, N2, N3) and one REM stage. The timing and depth of each stage vary across the night, but together they determine how well your body recovers, repairs and regenerates. When these stages are disrupted or shortened, it affects everything from memory and hormone regulation to mitochondrial repair and immune repair, hormonal balance and cellular recovery.

STAGE 1: LIGHT SLEEP

This is the transition phase – the first few minutes after you fall asleep. Brain waves begin to slow, though muscle tone and breathing remain similar to when you're awake. It's easy to wake from this stage, and most people cycle through it multiple times per night.

STAGE 2: MODERATE SLEEP

You disconnect more deeply from the outside world. Brain activity continues to slow, marked by brief bursts known as sleep spindles and K-complexes, which help protect sleep and play a key role in memory consolidation. During this stage your memories are processed and consolidated, much like a librarian organizing books in a massive library. Heart rate and body temperature drop. Stage 2 makes up the largest percentage of total sleep and lengthens with each cycle.

STAGE 3: DEEP SLEEP

This is the most restorative stage of non-REM sleep. The body repairs tissue and bone, builds muscle and strengthens the immune system. Growth hormone peaks, mitochondria enter a recovery mode and the glymphatic system activates to clear waste from the brain. Waking from Stage 3 often results in grogginess – and missing it can accelerate biological ageing. Deep sleep is most abundant in the first half of the night, so going to bed later reduces your total deep sleep, even if you sleep in.

STAGE 4: REM SLEEP

Rapid eye movement (REM) increases in length across the night. This is the stage where dreams occur – but more importantly, it's when your brain recalibrates neurotransmitters like serotonin and dopamine, which impact pleasure and motivation. Emotional processing, learning integration and memory organization happen here. Although breathing becomes irregular and brain activity spikes, your skeletal muscles are temporarily paralysed, preventing you from acting out dreams. Brain chemical balancing happens in this stage as well, which is why REM-sleep deprivation can mimic aspects of ADHD and emotional dysregulation.

You don't need to memorize these stages, but you do need to protect the full cycle. Skipping even one stage weakens the benefits of sleep. Late nights, alcohol and inconsistent schedules all fragment this rhythm. Aim to go to bed early enough to capture both deep Stage 3 sleep and the REM-rich cycles that occur later in the night – this is when your body repairs and your brain restores.

SLEEP DISRUPTORS: WHAT'S HIJACKING YOUR REST

A full seven to nine hours in bed doesn't necessarily translate to high-quality sleep. Your environment, behaviours and biology all influence the depth and stability of your sleep cycles. Below are some of the most common disruptors – and how they interfere with your body's ability to recover and build resilience.

LIGHT EXPOSURE AT NIGHT

Light – especially blue wavelengths from phones, laptops or overhead LEDs – suppresses melatonin, your body's sleep signal. Without sufficient melatonin, the circadian rhythm drifts off track, delaying sleep onset and shortening deep sleep. Even brief light exposure after sunset can reduce total melatonin by 50 per cent. Ideally, avoid screens and bright lighting in the one to two hours before bed or use red-shifted bulbs and blue light filters.

IRREGULAR SLEEP AND WAKE TIMES

Your circadian rhythm thrives on consistency. Sleeping in on weekends or shifting your bedtime by more than thirty to sixty minutes can desynchronize your internal clock – disrupting hormonal cycles, metabolism and body temperature regulation. Irregular schedules are also associated with lower sleep efficiency and reduced HRV. Aim to wake up and go to bed at roughly the same time every day, even on weekends.

BLOOD SUGAR INSTABILITY

Unstable blood glucose can trigger mid-night awakenings – especially between 2 and 4 a.m. High-carb meals or alcohol before bed can cause a spike-and-crash pattern that activates your stress response, jolting you awake. For people with insulin resistance, this is even more common. Aim to balance your blood sugar throughout the day with protein, healthy fats and fibre, and consider a small, balanced evening snack if you tend to wake hungry or anxious.

ALCOHOL & CAFFEINE

Alcohol fragments your sleep, increases night-time awakenings and suppresses REM – even in small amounts. Caffeine blocks adenosine, the neurotransmitter that builds sleep pressure. With a half-life of five to six hours, it can remain in your system long after your afternoon coffee. The sweet spot? Avoid caffeine after 2 p.m. and alcohol within two or three hours of bed.

CHRONIC INFLAMMATION & STRESS

Stress hormones like cortisol raise your heart rate and body temperature, blocking access to deep sleep. Cells that trigger inflammation have also been shown to impair REM and slow-wave sleep. And this isn't just about feeling stressed or experiencing anxiety. Systemic inflammation from poor gut health, overtraining or unresolved infections can fragment sleep even when your mind is calm. You may feel wired but tired, wake unrefreshed or need naps just to get through the day. Long term, this state reduces oxygen delivery to the brain, impairs glucose metabolism in the prefrontal cortex and undermines productivity, creativity and focus.

GENETICS: THE HIDDEN VARIABLE

Sometimes, sleep struggles run deeper than habits or environment – your genes may also be involved. Certain genetic variants like those affecting melatonin production, methylation or serotonin signalling can make it harder to fall or stay asleep. For example, people with MTHFR mutations may be more prone to anxiety or restlessness, which impacts sleep quality. And if you've ever felt wired but tired at night for no obvious reason, your DNA might be part of the picture.

Knowing your genetic tendencies can help you personalize your approach, whether it's prioritizing B-vitamin support, experimenting with 5-HTP (a precursor to melatonin) or syncing your schedule with your chronotype. Genes load the gun, but lifestyle pulls the trigger. While testing offers clarity, daily choices still make the biggest difference.

HOW TO IMPROVE YOUR SLEEP

When it comes to improving sleep, the goal is to remove friction – anything that blocks your body's natural ability to rest deeply. Your body is wired to sleep deeply when the right signals are in place. These evidence-based strategies help support the full architecture of sleep: from falling asleep faster to reaching deeper stages of recovery.

ANCHOR YOUR CIRCADIAN RHYTHM

Your circadian rhythm relies on strong cues to stay in sync. The most powerful ones? Light and timing. Get five to fifteen minutes of sunlight within an hour of waking – even on cloudy days. At night, dim your lights and avoid screens one to two hours before bed. Consistency matters just as much: go to bed and wake up at the same time every day, even on weekends. This stabilizes your hormone cycles, temperature rhythms and sleep depth.

SUPPORT BLOOD SUGAR STABILITY

Low or unstable blood glucose is a hidden driver of mid-sleep wakeups. Avoid high-glycaemic foods and alcohol in the evening. Instead, eat a protein-rich dinner with some complex carbohydrates (like whole grains, vegetables, or legumes) to support serotonin and melatonin production. Fibre intake is associated with getting more deep sleep at night, and one study found that eating a kiwi before bed helped people fall asleep faster and stay asleep longer. If you tend to wake up anxious or hungry at night, a small pre-bed snack with protein and slow carbs may help stabilize blood sugar and improve sleep continuity.

WIND DOWN YOUR NERVOUS SYSTEM

Your body won't sleep deeply if it's still in fight-or-flight mode. Create a thirty- to sixty-minute buffer before bed for wind-down: reading, journalling, light stretching or breathing exercises. A warm bath, infrared sauna or shower one to two hours before bed can also trigger thermoregulation: by bringing heat to the skin, your core temperature drops quicker, helping you fall asleep faster. If you tend to overthink, keep a notebook nearby and offload any to-do items before lying down.

OPTIMIZE YOUR SLEEP ENVIRONMENT

Light, sound and air all impact sleep depth. Use blackout curtains or an eye mask. Keep your room cool (ideally 16–19°C / 60–67°F) and quiet – or mask external sounds with white or brown noise. Use a HEPA filter to reduce allergens and improve air quality. And don't overlook the visual environment: visual clutter is cognitive clutter. A clean, calm bedroom sends a signal that it's time to rest, not think.

USE TARGETED SUPPLEMENT SUPPORT

If sleep remains fragmented even with strong habits, targeted supplements may help regulate neurotransmitters and nervous system tone. Always consult a healthcare provider before starting a new protocol. Some low-risk options to consider:

- Magnesium glycinate or bisglycinate (200–400 mg): calms the nervous system and can help you fall asleep more quickly.

- L-theanine (100–200 mg): an amino acid that promotes relaxation without drowsiness.

- 5-HTP (50–100 mg): a serotonin precursor that can support melatonin production, especially for those with low mood or disrupted sleep onset.

- Glycine (3 g): may help lower core body temperature and improve sleep quality.

Going to bed at the same time every night is one of the simplest ways to optimise your circadian rhythm.

TRACK YOUR SLEEP

Not all sleep is equal, and the way you feel in the morning doesn't always tell the full story. Tracking your sleep gives you insight into the patterns, depth and disruptions that might be impacting your recovery and energy. It also helps you connect the dots between lifestyle habits and biological outcomes.

WHAT TO TRACK

Most wearable devices estimate the time you spend in different sleep stages and offer sleep scores based on factors like:

- Sleep onset latency (how long it takes you to fall asleep).

- Total sleep duration (how long you spent asleep).

- Sleep efficiency (how much of your time in bed was spent asleep).

- Wake episodes (how often and how long you were awake).

These trends matter more than the day-to-day fluctuations. If you consistently see short deep sleep, fragmented REM or low total duration, your body isn't completing full recovery cycles. And over time, that catches up to you.

THE POWER OF HRV

Heart rate variability (HRV) is one of the most sensitive indicators of recovery, stress and nervous system balance. Higher HRV generally reflects greater adaptability and resilience. Low HRV, especially when paired with poor sleep, signals that your system is under strain from inflammation, overtraining, blood sugar dysregulation or emotional stress. The best time to measure HRV is overnight or just after waking. Use the baseline average over weeks – not isolated numbers – to assess whether your habits are helping or harming your body's ability to reset. Tools like Oura Ring, WHOOP, Apple Watch and Garmin can track this automatically, but even without wearables, a consistent morning pulse check and subjective energy rating can give you clues.

DON'T OBSESS, OBSERVE

Sleep data is most helpful when it leads to better self-awareness, not stress. If you find yourself chasing perfect scores, zoom out. The real goal is consistency, not perfection. Your body will tell you if something's working long before your app does.

WORK WITH YOUR CHRONOTYPE, NOT AGAINST IT

Ever wonder why some people bounce out of bed at 6 a.m. and others feel most alive at midnight? You may be programmed this way. Your chronotype reflects your genetically influenced sleep–wake preference, or when your body naturally wants to rise, focus, wind down and sleep.

Chronotypes exist on a spectrum from early birds to night owls. Trying to force yourself into a rhythm that doesn't match your wiring – like waking at 5 a.m. when your body prefers 8 a.m. – creates ongoing misalignment with your biology. This mismatch leads to sleep inertia, mood imbalances, poor focus and low resilience, even if you're technically 'getting enough sleep'.

To identify your chronotype, try tracking your natural sleep–wake patterns during a period without external obligations (holidays, weekends or flexible days). Pay attention to:

- When you naturally get sleepy.
- When you feel most focused and productive.
- When your energy dips or peaks throughout the day.

You can also explore tools like the Morningness–Eveningness Questionnaire (MEQ) or the Munich Chronotype Questionnaire (MCTQ) to get a more structured insight. Most importantly, once you know your rhythm – protect it. Align your bedtime, meals and focus time accordingly. That's where real recovery can happen.

But what if you *still* can't sleep? If you've implemented the suggestions in this chapter with consistency and patience, given them time to work, yet still find yourself tossing and turning, it may be time to dig deeper.

Chronic insomnia or excessive daytime fatigue can be signs of an underlying sleep disorder. A health professional can help guide next steps, such as a sleep study (polysomnography) or therapies like CBT-I (cognitive behavioural therapy for insomnia), which is the gold-standard treatment for long-term sleep issues. Sleep problems can also signal deeper imbalances in the body. Conditions like arthritis, chronic pain, depression, anxiety and even gut dysfunction are linked to disrupted sleep – and many of them share a common root: inflammation.

Even one night of insufficient sleep can alter the expression of over 700 genes, many involved in inflammation, stress response, immunity, metabolism and repair. Over time, this creates a state of biological chaos – heightening reactivity, depleting resilience and accelerating cellular ageing.

Sleep is an active healing process that touches every system in your body, and it's one of the most powerful, free forms of preventative medicine we have. Reframing your relationship with sleep and prioritizing it on a consistent basis is a radical act of self-love. The results? More energy, clearer thinking, better moods, stronger immune function and a body that feels like it's working with you, not against you.

CHAPTER SUMMARY

Sleep isn't optional. It's fundamental. Every night, your body repairs mitochondria, balances hormones, clears brain waste, resets insulin sensitivity and recalibrates your immune system. It does this on a rhythm, and when that rhythm breaks, the fallout ripples through every cell, organ and system.

Modern life disrupts that rhythm daily. But the good news is: your biology is responsive. You can restore alignment with surprisingly simple strategies.

HOW TO SLEEP TO LIVE LONGER

- Wake at the same time each day: even weekends. This is your anchor.

- Get sunlight within sixty minutes of waking: light resets your biological clock faster than any supplement.

- Use blue-light blockers or red-tinted bulbs in the evening to protect your melatonin levels.

- Calm your nervous system before bed with magnesium, journalling, a weighted blanket or a warm bath.

- Move during the day, wind down at night: circadian rhythms depend on contrast.

- Limit screens and mental stimulation in the evening — choose wind-down over scroll-down.

- If sleep remains fragmented, consider testing for sleep-disrupting imbalances (inflammation, hormone shifts, methylation issues) or speaking with a provider.

Sleep isn't about perfection. It's about rhythm, consistency and recovery. The more aligned you are with your natural patterns, the more clearly you'll think, the more deeply you'll heal and the younger your body will feel. Prioritize sleep not because it's easy, but because everything else gets easier when you do.

'When chaos is all around you, the wisest choice is to create peace within you.'

Yung Pueblo

Poet, meditator and speaker

THINK

There's no longevity without a calm, adaptive mind. Your thoughts, your stress response, your daily habits of attention – they shape your biology in real time. Western medicine tends to separate mental and physical health, but your nervous system doesn't. It's always listening, always reacting, always regulating ... or failing to. You can eat the best diet, surround yourself with the best people and follow the smartest workouts. But if you're not working on your mindset and doing the things that set your soul on fire – real happiness and deep health will stay just out of reach.

In this chapter, we'll explore how your mind influences your mitochondria, your hormones and your ability to recover from stress. The goal isn't to avoid stress, it's to build resilience to it. We'll look at the science behind this resilience and give you practical ways to train your nervous system, not just for peace of mind but for a longer, more vibrant life.

WHEN STRESS IS THE PROBLEM – RESILIENCE IS THE SOLUTION

You often hear stress spoken about like it's the enemy – but that's only half true. It's not the presence of stress that damages health. It's the absence of proper recovery. Stress is a biological signal. It mobilizes energy, sharpens your focus and helps you rise to the occasion. In fact, acute stressors – short, time-bound challenges like exercise, cold plunges or breath-holds – can actually benefit your mitochondria by triggering adaptive repair. These hormetic stressors make your cells more efficient, your brain more resilient and your lifespan potentially longer.

Issues arise with chronic stress when there's no clear beginning or end, and no opportunity to reset. Constant mental noise, emotional suppression, too much screen time, too little rest – these keep your nervous system on high alert. That's when your mitochondria start to falter. Cortisol remains elevated, inflammation builds, blood sugar regulation goes haywire and long-term wear and tear accelerates ageing from the inside out.

Resilience isn't about avoiding stress altogether. It's about training your nervous system to recover well. And that starts with understanding how to recognize dysregulation and build daily practices that bring you back to balance, again and again.

WHEN YOUR NERVOUS SYSTEM IS STUCK IN OVERDRIVE

When your nervous system is in balance, you feel grounded, calm and connected. Your digestion works. Your thoughts flow clearly. Your energy feels steady. But when your body gets stuck in a survival response – like fight, flight, freeze or fawn – everything changes. You might feel anxious, restless, withdrawn or like you're always on edge. Rather than any character flaws, these are biological responses from a system that hasn't learned how to return to safety.

Over time, being stuck in a survival state affects your whole body. Your mitochondria produce less energy. Your hormones shift, your immune system weakens, your sleep gets disrupted and decision-making feels harder. You may feel wired but tired – alert, but exhausted. Your HRV drops, a signal that your resilience is wearing thin.

It's easy to start identifying with these states. You might think, *I'm just not a relaxed person*, or *this is just who I am*. But the reality is, it's what your nervous system has learned to do to protect you. Sometimes the stressor is long gone, but your body still holds on. Unfinished stress responses stay stuck in your physiology, like alarms that never get turned off. That's why certain sounds, smells or situations can set off big reactions: your body remembers, even when your mind doesn't.

Regulation isn't about being calm all the time. It's about knowing how to come home to yourself. With practice, you can teach your body that it's safe to let go. You don't need to earn safety – you just need to remember how it feels.

THE BODY KEEPS THE SCORE

Unprocessed emotions don't just disappear: they settle into the tissues of the body. You've probably felt it before: the tight chest during grief, the lump in your throat when you hold back tears, the tension in your jaw when you're angry but can't express it. These aren't metaphors or random experiences. They're biological signals that your nervous system didn't get to complete. This is the essence of the mind–body connection: what you don't resolve mentally, your body will try to hold. Trauma expert Dr Bessel van der Kolk called this 'the body keeping the score'. And it does – in your fascia, your posture, your breath, your digestion and your energy levels.

The fascia, your body's connective tissue matrix, plays a surprising role here. It's more than just structural scaffolding – it stores emotional tension and past trauma, sometimes for decades. This is the principle behind somatic release techniques like those used by wellness and bodywork centre Human Garage, where physical manipulation of fascia can lead to spontaneous emotional release: laughter, tears or even vivid memories. When you release the tension in the tissue, you often unlock the emotion that got stuck there. These stored stress patterns can shape how you move, breathe and relate to the world, often without our conscious awareness. Over time, they contribute to chronic pain, fatigue, anxiety or even the feeling of being disconnected from your body.

Healing starts with awareness. Instead of pushing through or numbing out, your body needs permission to *feel* – safely, gently and without judgement. When you give it that space, you're not just healing emotions, you're restoring flow, resilience and vitality at the cellular level.

The brain isn't fixed at adulthood.
You can reshape it at any age
with the right tools.

HOW TO BUILD RESILIENCE: REGULATING YOUR NERVOUS SYSTEM

Your nervous system is constantly scanning your environment to determine whether you're safe. When it feels overwhelmed, you might feel anxious, short-tempered, shut down or scattered. When it feels supported, you feel calm, grounded and able to respond instead of react. What you eat, watch, listen to, scroll through and surround yourself with becomes the input that either soothes or stimulates your internal state. Ask yourself: *Is this nourishing me or depleting me?* That question alone can help you reset your internal compass.

Simple practices like mindfulness, meditation or even just three minutes of slow breathing can shift your body into a parasympathetic, healing state. A few of the fastest ways to do this are listed on the following pages.

- Breathwork: try a 4:8 pattern – inhale for four seconds, exhale for eight seconds. This extended exhale signals safety to your brain and activates your vagus nerve.

- Vagal toning: gentle stimulation of the vagus nerve (like humming, gargling, splashing cold water on your face or singing) helps regulate your nervous system and reduce inflammation.

- Nature time: being in nature lowers cortisol and boosts mitochondrial health. It also reminds your body what safety feels like.

- Acts of service: helping others lowers stress hormones and increases oxytocin. Kindness isn't only a virtue; it's a longevity practice.

- Purpose and mindset: starting your day with intention – *today will be a good day* – changes the way your brain filters experience. A sense of meaning and purpose has been linked to longer life, reduced dementia risk and greater resilience.

- Digital boundaries: reduce overstimulation by limiting screen time, decluttering your space and turning off notifications. Your nervous system isn't built for constant input.

You don't need a silent retreat to feel regulated. You need small, consistent practices that remind your body it's safe – and that *you're* in charge.

CREATE STRONG SENSORY BOUNDARIES

Stress is often thought of as emotional, but sensory input plays a major role in how regulated or overwhelmed your nervous system feels. Constant exposure to loud sounds, harsh lighting, fast scrolling or even just visual clutter can keep your system in a low-level state of vigilance. Over time, this overstimulation adds up – draining energy, disrupting sleep and making it harder to focus or feel at ease.

Creating strong sensory boundaries is one of the most powerful, underutilized tools for nervous system health. That might mean dimming the lights at night, turning off your phone an hour before bed, organizing your space to reduce visual mess or choosing calm, quiet environments when you need to recover. Your nervous system doesn't just need motivation. It needs *margin*. Giving yourself space to feel safe, still and internally quiet is a daily gift and a biological necessity.

COME BACK TO YOURSELF: RITUAL, GRATITUDE AND PLAY

Your nervous system is deeply pattern-based. When life feels unpredictable, structure becomes your medicine. Even something as simple as lighting a candle at the same time each evening can serve as a cue for your body to exhale. Daily rituals like morning walks, shared meals and consistent bedtimes can create a sense of internal safety too.

Gratitude is also more than just a nice idea. It's a cellular intervention. A meta-analysis of sixty-four gratitude intervention trials found consistent improvements in mental health – including lower anxiety and depression, more positive emotions and better life satisfaction. On the physical side, gratitude practices have been linked to reduced markers of inflammation and improved sleep quality.

And then there's play – the most underrated healing tool of all. When was the last time you did something just for fun? Not for productivity, not for progress. Just for joy. What did you love doing as a child before you were told to 'grow up'? What have you always wanted to try but haven't given yourself permission to start? Play isn't frivolous. It sparks neuroplasticity, increases mitochondrial health and reconnects you to vitality.

Let yourself build sandcastles. Paint with your fingers. Learn the drums. Try improv. Be a beginner. Because this, more than any smoothie or supplement, is what keeps you alive inside.

EXPLORE PSYCHOSOMATIC HEALING

It's incredible to be living in a time where science is innovating personalized vaccines to fight cancer, regenerating organs inside the body and decoding the genome in real time. And yet, mystery symptoms persist. Chronic pain, fatigue, gut issues, muscle tension. Often, diagnostic tests come back 'normal', but the symptoms are very real.

This disconnect is what gave rise to the study of psychosomatic medicine. This practice does not suggest the symptoms are imagined but recognizes that the mind and body are in constant dialogue. There is substantial evidence supporting the existence of psychosomatic diseases, which could, in part, explain this phenomenon. Studies demonstrate how psychological stress can lead to physical symptoms such as headaches, indigestion, constipation and more.

Dr John Sarno, a rehabilitation physician at New York University, became known for identifying a condition he called Tension Myositis Syndrome (TMS). He believed that unconscious emotional stress – rage, fear, grief – could manifest physically by reducing blood flow to muscles and nerves, resulting in real pain.

A more widely accepted and clinically grounded perspective can be found in somatic therapies like Babette Rothschild's Somatic Trauma Therapy, which works with the autonomic nervous system to process unresolved stress stored in the body. These approaches suggest that true healing doesn't always begin with medication or surgery; it begins with awareness.

MEDITATE

Meditation in itself is a biological upgrade. At its core, meditation is the practice of focused awareness, training your attention on something simple – like the breath, a sound or a physical sensation – while noticing (without judgement) when your mind wanders. Your goal shouldn't be to stop your thoughts but to relate to them differently. Numerous studies have demonstrated that regular meditation can lead to significant reductions in stress, anxiety and depression.

However, the advantages of meditation extend far beyond mental health benefits. Research has unveiled *physiological* changes linked to consistent meditation practice, too. For example, one of the most striking findings is its potential to lower blood pressure, a critical factor in heart health. Meditation also supports mitochondrial function and, according to emerging research, can increase the number of circulating stem cells, mobilizing them from your own bone marrow into the bloodstream, where they support regeneration. Meditation may also improve immune function in individuals who practise it regularly. Research has also shown that meditation may counteract stress-induced telomere shortening, a process in which the protective caps at the ends of chromosomes (telomeres) gradually shrink over time. Telomere shortening is associated with ageing-related diseases, as it can lead to cellular dysfunction and reduced ability to regenerate. Finally, an eight-week meditation study revealed significant changes in the expression of 172 genes involved in regulating inflammation, circadian rhythms and glucose metabolism.

Crucially, meditation shifts your nervous system out of fight-or-flight and into rest-and-repair – the state where healing happens. Over time, it strengthens brain regions tied to memory, focus and emotional regulation. And beyond biology, meditation builds awareness. You begin to recognize your patterns, your inner dialogue and your stress responses with more clarity.

MEDITATION MADE SIMPLE

Integrating an effective meditation practice into your daily life doesn't require hours of spare time, special equipment or a serene mountain retreat. You can start with just ten minutes a day, as research shows this is enough to ease symptoms of depression and anxiety, and even make you more likely to exercise, eat well and sleep better.

If you're new to meditation, you might find it helpful to begin with a guided practice. Popular apps like Calm, Waking Up, Headspace or the free app Medito offer a variety of short, beginner-friendly sessions that focus on stress relief, relaxation and better sleep. Over time, as you grow more comfortable, you can experiment with meditating on your own. Mindfulness meditation can be as simple as sitting quietly, closing your eyes, focusing on your breath and gently observing your thoughts — without judgement or the need to change anything.

You can also try incorporating mindfulness into your daily activities. For example, mindful walking involves paying close attention to each step, the sensations in your body and the rhythm of your breath as you move. Even mundane tasks like washing the dishes or drinking tea can become a form of meditation when done mindfully.

AVOID 'DOPAMINE OVERLOAD'

Dopamine is often called the feel-good chemical, but that's an oversimplification. As much as dopamine is about pleasure, it's also about pursuit. Dopamine fuels motivation, craving and anticipation. It's the chemical behind the urge to scroll when bored, snack when stressed or refresh your inbox for no reason at all. In a balanced system, dopamine spikes in anticipation of a reward and then dips once the experience ends. That dip is part of homeostasis: your brain's effort to stay in balance. But in today's world of constant stimulation, that balance is under siege.

Social media, streaming platforms, online shopping, porn and even hyper-palatable foods are all designed to hijack your dopamine system. They deliver quick hits without effort, bypassing the natural friction that once limited overindulgence. In evolutionary terms, our ancestors had to work hard for every reward. Now, dopamine is available on demand, 24/7. This constant stimulation keeps the limbic system – the emotional, reactive part of the brain – dominant, while sidelining the prefrontal cortex, the part responsible for impulse control, decision-making and long-term planning. Over time, this imbalance can chip away at your ability to tolerate discomfort, delay gratification and solve real-world problems. It also contributes to rising rates of anxiety, depression and digital burnout.

The solution isn't to eliminate dopamine but rather to reset your sensitivity to it. Psychiatrist Dr Anna Lembke, author of *Dopamine Nation*, recommends a temporary fast from your biggest dopamine triggers. That could mean twenty-four hours without your phone or thirty days without social media, shopping apps or added sugar.

The goal isn't permanent abstinence. It's space. Space to rebuild your baseline and reconnect with simple pleasures that aren't hijacked by addictive design. Once the fast is complete, reintroduce your habit with intention. Add friction. Remove devices from your bedroom. Use airplane mode during certain hours. Make the habit a choice – not a reflex. As Dr Lembke puts it: 'It's easier to go from abstinence to moderation than from overconsumption to moderation.'

HEALTHY DOPAMINE FIXES

Once you create space from overstimulating habits, your brain starts to reset. These practices help you get your 'dopamine fix' in healthier ways, for example:

- Phone-free first hour: delay screen time for at least sixty minutes after waking. This protects your brain's natural dopamine rhythm and prevents an early spike that can leave you feeling scattered all day.

- Walk before the screen: replace morning scrolling with movement — ideally outdoors. A ten-minute walk boosts dopamine naturally, balances cortisol and sets the tone for clearer thinking.

- Dopamine detox blocks: schedule thirty to sixty minutes of intentional low-stimulation time each day – no screens, no multitasking. Giving your brain space to be bored is a powerful way to rewire reward pathways.

- Create a dopamine menu: list healthy, high-dopamine habits (like weight training or singing) and low-dopamine anchors (like tea or journalling). Start your day with natural sources before layering in digital ones.

- Protein-rich breakfast: dopamine is built from tyrosine, found in protein-rich foods. A breakfast of eggs, Greek yoghurt or chia pudding supports mood, motivation and cognitive clarity.

- Listen to music: create a playlist of your favourite songs and have it ready to play when you feel you need a boost. Listening to the music you love will make your brain release dopamine.

LEARN FOR LIFE

You didn't come to earth just to survive. You came to create, express and grow. Learning isn't just about brain health, it's about discovering who you are and what you're here to do.

Studies show that engaging in new, challenging experiences helps preserve cognitive function and build resilience as you age. But beyond the biological benefits, learning invites you to reconnect with curiosity, confidence and self-expression – the raw materials of purpose.

The brain thrives on novelty. So does the soul. Whether you're learning a new language, starting pottery, fixing your bike or reading something that challenges your worldview, it all adds up. You're not just building neural pathways – you're building *yourself*.

NEUROPLASTICITY IN PRACTICE

New experiences help us remember what we're capable of. Try something that stretches you mentally, creatively or emotionally. It might be:

- Learning a new skill you've always put off.

- Making something with your hands.

- Challenging yourself to see a familiar topic in a new light.

You don't need hours. Just fifteen minutes a few times a week with something that sparks genuine interest can be enough. Follow what excites you, even if it feels small or strange. Growth is rarely linear, but it's always worth it.

THINK YOURSELF YOUNG

Your body responds to your belief system. If you speak to yourself like you believe your life is full of vitality, purpose and joy – your biology will start to follow. And this isn't just mindset talk. In 1981, Harvard psychologist Dr Ellen Langer ran a now-famous experiment known as the 'counterclockwise study'. Eight men in their late seventies and early eighties lived for a week in a monastery recreated to look, sound and feel like it was 1959. They wore their younger clothes, discussed current events from that year and were instructed to think, speak and act as if they were decades younger. By the end of the week, they showed measurable improvements in strength, vision, hearing, posture and memory. In other words, their bodies began to respond to the mindset of youth.

The results have since been echoed in follow-up studies, including a BBC replication where participants regained lost mobility, and in broader research a Yale study found that people who held positive views on ageing lived an average of 7.5 years longer than those who didn't. Subjective age, or how old you *feel*, has measurable effects on both lifespan and healthspan. But this isn't simply pretending you're twenty-five. It's about rejecting the cultural conditioning that says your best years are behind you. It's about embodying vitality, curiosity and possibility at any age.

Sergey Young, longevity investor and author of *The Science and Technology of Growing Young*, shares that once he began viewing himself as a thirty-something aiming to live to 200, everything shifted. He started moving more, taking stairs two at a time and feeling mentally sharper. A simple mindset shift produced real changes in energy and behaviour. Examples are everywhere. Tao Porchon-Lynch began competitive ballroom dancing in her eighties and performed on *America's Got Talent* at ninety-six. Grandma Moses picked up painting in her late seventies and became one of the most celebrated folk artists in American history. These aren't outliers – they're reminders.

> Age is not a barrier. It's a container you get to fill with whatever you want. So if there's something you've been putting off because you feel 'too old', consider this your invitation.

CHAPTER SUMMARY

Your mind isn't just along for the ride – it's shaping your biology in real time. Your thoughts and emotional patterns influence how you age, how you heal and how fully you live. This chapter looks at the ripple effects of stress and mindset, not to 'fix' the mind but to work with it as a powerful tool for longevity and vitality.

- Long-term stress wears the body down. Practices like breathwork, meditation and nervous system retraining help restore your ability to bounce back.

- Emotional pain often finds its way into the body. The more you explore your internal world, the more clues you uncover about your physical symptoms.

- Resetting your relationship with dopamine – how you chase it, how you soothe – can shift everything from your focus to your mood.

- How you *feel* about ageing affects how you experience it. People who feel younger often tend to live younger – and longer.

- Staying curious, trying new things and learning about yourself – these are underrated longevity tools. They keep your brain flexible and your confidence strong. Self-compassion, curiosity, presence: they aren't soft skills. They're some of the most powerful tools you have for staying well.

'The meaning of life is to find your gift. The purpose of life is to give it away.'

Pablo Picasso

Artist

LIVE

There's a quiet turning point in many people's lives. It might even feel like a whisper. Maybe it shows up when you're sitting on a train, wondering what you're racing toward. Maybe it stirs after a big achievement that doesn't feel as satisfying as you thought it would. Or maybe it shows up in the in-between moments: a conversation, a heartbreak, a sunrise, when you realize something inside you is longing for more.

When was the last time you woke up excited? Not just 'I have a lot to do' – but excitement that you feel in your bones. The kind that makes you feel grateful to be alive and grounded, even if life isn't going perfectly. Maybe it's been a while, and that's OK. You've been moving fast, doing the things you thought you were supposed to – chasing productivity, success or security – only to realize you've lost touch with something much more essential: purpose. Our purpose isn't something to find in a book or check off a list. It's something that lives in your body. And your purpose isn't what you do, it's *who you are*.

It doesn't always come with a grand plan, but it's the clarity to see how every single moment was a perfect stepping stone to make you the person you are today. It's about living with intention, reconnecting with your values and creating a life that's not only meaningful but feels that way too.

And science now echoes what many have intuitively felt: living with purpose keeps us alive – literally. In a study of nearly 7,000 adults over fifty, those who felt the least sense of purpose were far more likely to die from any cause than those who felt deeply connected to their 'why'. The takeaway? Having a strong reason to get up in the morning might just help you live longer. Purpose may be as vital to our health as exercise or diet, acting as a protective factor against physical and emotional decline. You may be able to add years to your life simply by engaging with meaningful pursuits.

But how do we discover our purpose? In today's world, it's easier than ever to stay busy and harder than ever to stay fulfilled. Unsurprisingly, studies show that many of us are increasingly less happy. Global depression rates have been climbing significantly in the past thirty years, with one in six adults in the UK experiencing health problems such as depression or anxiety. We've never been so out of touch with our minds, bodies and souls, chasing after things that supposedly bring fulfilment, like a bigger pay cheque, a nicer car or a better home. One of the longest-running studies in the world – The Harvard Study of Adult Development – found that what truly keeps us happy and healthy as we age isn't wealth or status. It's the quality of our close relationships.

Strong, emotionally supportive connections not only improve our mood, they shape our long-term wellbeing more than any external marker of success. And while the pursuit of material goods was linked to lower life satisfaction, participants who focused on personal growth and emotional connection reported better sleep, stronger mental health and a higher quality of life.

Another large-scale study, tracking over 12,000 adults, found that a strong sense of purpose was linked to a 46 per cent lower risk of death, better sleep, lower depression and decreased loneliness, as well as higher levels of optimism. In other words, living with purpose doesn't just feel good – it may be one of the most protective things we can do for our long-term health.

FIND YOUR IKIGAI

Ikigai is a Japanese concept that blends two words: *iki* meaning 'to live', and *gai* meaning 'reason', and literally translates into 'a reason to live.' It's often visualized as the intersection between what you love, what you're good at, what the world needs and what you can be paid for. While some versions of the framework leave out the last piece – compensation – it's not because earning money is unimportant. It's because ikigai isn't meant to only be used as a career plan, as it's much more than that. It's the unique way you're meant to show up in the world, guided by what brings you joy, purpose and meaning.

It doesn't have to be grand to be meaningful. As Paulo Coelho wrote, purpose isn't found – it's remembered. Often, it's something we've carried within us for a long time, waiting to be noticed. Your ikigai can also shift over time. As you grow and change, so might the way you live it out. What matters is not doing more but feeling more deeply connected to what matters.

Research shows that people with a strong sense of purpose tend to live longer, have healthier hearts and have a better quality of life. When you live with intention without having to have all the answers, you are intuitively led to how you can give, create and connect.

MAPPING YOUR MEANING: AN IKIGAI EXPLORATION

You don't find your ikigai in one perfect moment. You live into it, choice by choice, year by year. It's not a destination, it's a direction. And it often begins with questions. Take a quiet moment. Put your hand on your heart, then gently ask:

- What brings me alive, even if no one notices?

- What have people always come to me for?

- What have I always wanted to try but told myself I was too late, too busy or not good enough?

- What breaks my heart, and how can I help heal the world from this?

- Where did life ask me to grow and how did that growth change what matters to me?

- What does the world need that I feel drawn to offer?

- How could this become sustainable, for my energy, my spirit and my livelihood?

Remember, purpose isn't just what you're passionate about but rather what you can be devoted to. While what excites you is important, it's just as meaningful to be willing to show up for others – with presence, empathy and hope. Let your answers unfold without pressure. You might write, voicenote, collage or simply reflect. You might even create a quiet space, a time each week to reconnect with what truly matters. Every 'yes' to your purpose is also a 'no' to distraction – and that is a sacred act.

How will you know when you've found your ikigai? Ikigai isn't usually something you stumble into in a single life-changing moment. It's something you grow into intentionally by paying attention to what brings you energy, peace and a sense of meaningful contribution. You may not always feel joyful – but you'll feel grounded. Sometimes, purpose feels like showing up when it's hard, staying committed to what matters and feeling the deep sense of resonance that comes from living in integrity. And remember, your ikigai doesn't have to be your job. In a 2010 survey of 2,000 Japanese adults, only 31 per cent said their ikigai was related to work. Sometimes it's a role you play in your community, a creative practice or simply the way you show up for the people you love.

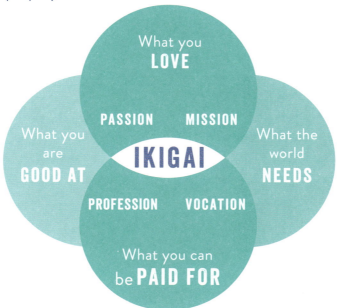

LIVE BY YOUR VALUES

Living a long, meaningful life doesn't begin with goals. It begins with values: the inner compass that guides your decisions, shapes your relationships and helps you stay rooted when life gets uncertain. Your values are more than just what you believe in, they're what you honour through your actions. And the more clearly you know them, the easier it becomes to live with integrity, to make aligned choices – even when things don't go as planned.

Values are deeply personal. For some, it's creativity or honesty. For others, it's community, adventure or peace. There's no right answer, only what's true for *you*. But without defining them, it's easy to get swept into decisions that don't reflect who you are.

Take a moment to reflect:

- What qualities do I admire most in others?
- What energizes me, and what drains me?
- What do I want people to feel when they're around me?

If you're not sure where to begin, think about three to five words from the list below that feel most important to you right now. Let them be your north star – not as something to *perfect* but to *practise*.

CREATIVITY

PLAYFULNESS

HONESTY

SIMPLICITY

JOY

INTEGRITY

KINDNESS

CURIOSITY

PRESENCE

SERVICE

COMPASSION

WISDOM

ADVENTURE

JUSTICE

PEACE

SPIRITUALITY

DISCIPLINE

GROWTH

COURAGE

AUTHENTICITY

FREEDOM

COMMUNITY

LOYALTY

BEAUTY

RESILIENCE

LOVE WELL: THE POWER OF PARTNERSHIP

Before we talk about relationships with others, we must first zoom in on the one you have with yourself. Living in alignment with your values – knowing who you are and what matters most – is one of the most protective, calming forces you can create for your nervous system. When your inner world is steady, it becomes easier to build partnerships that are rooted in trust, reciprocity and mutual growth. Your values become the compass for who and how you love, not just romantically but across all areas of life.

When talking about long-term partnership, the science is clear: healthy, committed love can be profoundly healing. Research has shown that those in long-term relationships often experience less depression, recover more quickly from illness and even live longer. One study showed that married people were half as likely to develop heart disease, and more likely to survive if they did. The presence of a steady partner – someone who knows your moods, your rhythms and your milestones – can ease the path through stress, medical treatments and everyday life.

There's even evidence that physical affection – like giving or receiving a massage, cuddling or making love – boosts oxytocin, the love hormone. This hormone can help reduce anxiety, lower stress and even improve mental wellbeing. Oxytocin may also have anti-ageing properties, reducing oxidative stress, mitigating chronic inflammation and promoting cellular regeneration. Some research suggests that men may benefit physically from marriage, while women benefit more emotionally, but only when the relationship is high-quality. A partnership built on tension or misalignment can add more stress than it relieves.

If you are in a relationship, the invitation is to nurture it intentionally. Communicate often, laugh together, move your bodies, share your meals and hold space for each other's dreams. And if you're single, know this: you haven't missed the window. The oldest bride on record was 102. The oldest groom, 103. And in the meantime, building a life of meaning, values and friendship is already medicine.

MAKE FRIENDS

One study found that having close social ties can increase your survival rate by 50 per cent. Another study revealed that loneliness is just as harmful to your health as smoking fifteen cigarettes a day. And the science goes deeper. UCLA researcher Dr Steven Cole found that certain genes tied to social connection also influence immune activity. In both humans and rhesus monkeys, social isolation triggered these genes to increase inflammation and suppress white blood cell production – making the body more vulnerable to illness and even tumour growth. In contrast, feeling socially supported helps your body stay more resilient.

But good relationships don't just happen. They require intention. Reaching out regularly, whether through texts, calls or ideally face to face, can help maintain bonds. Rituals like weekly dinners, long walks or even ten-minute check-ins can create a rhythm of closeness.

Volunteering, joining a community group or simply saying yes to more social invitations can also open doors to new, values-aligned friendships. One study even found that people who volunteered were 24 per cent more likely to join community groups or organizations – naturally expanding their support networks.

And remember: it's not about how many people you know but how known you feel. Real friendship takes time. Researchers at the University of Kansas found that it takes approximately forty to sixty hours together to go from acquaintance to casual friend; eighty to 100 hours to become true friends; and over 200 hours to form a deep, lasting bond. So give it time, because friendship is one of the most powerful forms of medicine we have.

GET A PET

There's something deeply healing about being needed – not for your achievements but simply for your presence. That's one of the quiet gifts of caring for a pet. In return they offer comfort, routine and an unspoken bond that anchors us through life's highs and lows. Research shows that pet owners experience less stress, lower rates of depression and even improved heart health. In fact, one study found that dog ownership is associated with a 24 per cent lower risk of all-cause mortality (meaning death from any cause). Part of this is physical – dogs get us outside and moving, rain or shine. But much of it is emotional. Pets can lower blood pressure levels, reduce cortisol and provide a steady source of companionship that buffers against loneliness. Even watching fish swim in an aquarium has been shown to promote relaxation.

For older adults especially, pets can offer routine, connection and a sense of purpose – three powerful ingredients for healthy ageing. But you don't need to adopt a pet to feel the benefits. Offer to walk a neighbour's dog, volunteer at a shelter or pet-sit for a friend. The simple act of tending to another living thing is a great way to live young, and a great reminder to tend to yourself as well.

GROW SOMETHING GREEN

Caring for a plant might seem like a small act, but its impact runs deep. After being surrounded by screens and artificial light, reconnecting with something alive and growing can bring surprising calm. It's a reminder that even the simplest forms of care can shift our biology. Plants do more than brighten a room. They purify the air, reduce toxins like formaldehyde and benzene and even boost oxygen levels – especially varieties like aloe vera and snake plants, which continue releasing oxygen at night. Some plants, like the areca palm or peace lily, are particularly good at filtering harmful volatile organic compounds (VOCs) from furniture and cleaning products.

But the most profound benefits might be felt rather than seen. Research shows that interacting with plants – watering, pruning or just sitting near them – lowers cortisol levels and supports better blood pressure regulation. Simply adding greenery to a workspace improved productivity by 15 per cent, reduced mental fatigue and enhanced focus. Another study found that plants may help calm the nervous system and bring the body into a more parasympathetic (relaxed) state.

LAUGH MORE

Turns out, the old saying 'laughter is the best medicine' has some serious scientific backup. In a study of over 17,000 adults in Japan, those who laughed daily had a lower risk of death from any cause. Another study looked at people across different age groups – from sixty-somethings to centenarians – and found that the oldest among them laughed the most often. Even Jeanne Calment, a French woman who lived to 122, swore that her long life came down to one thing: keeping a sense of humour. 'I think I'll die laughing,' she once said.

But laughter does more than just brighten your mood. It lowers cortisol, the stress hormone, and boosts the release of endorphins, our body's natural painkillers. Laughing also increases oxygen intake and circulation, which benefits your heart and supports overall vitality. In short: laughing isn't just joyful, it's biological. Whether it's a goofy moment with a loved one, your favourite comedy or an unexpected giggle, every laugh sends a ripple of healing through your body. Make room for more of them, and they might just help you live longer – and certainly better.

GIGGLE THERAPY

Laughter isn't just good for your health, it's one of the fastest ways to boost connection, ease stress and brighten your day. Here are a few playful ways to invite more joy into your routine:

- Watch your favourite comedians, light-hearted films or silly YouTube clips that never fail to make you laugh.

- Share jokes, memes or funny observations with friends and co-workers. A little levity goes a long way.

- Try games that spark laughter, especially ones that involve creativity or a bit of friendly chaos.

- Take a laughter yoga class – they combine breathing exercises and forced laughter (which usually turns real) to help you tap into joy and ease.

- When you can, laugh at your own missteps. Embracing imperfection with humour can turn stress into softness.

Whether it's a deep belly laugh or a quiet snort at your phone, every giggle counts.

BE GRATEFUL

Gratitude is a physiological state that reshapes how your body handles stress, ageing and even disease. In a study of nearly 50,000 older women, those with higher levels of gratitude had significantly lower rates of mortality. Why? Because gratitude shifts the entire nervous system towards calm. It's linked to better sleep, lower blood pressure and fewer doctor visits. Grateful people also tend to move more, stress less and feel more satisfied with life overall.

But gratitude isn't just about listing what's going well. It's also about perspective. Sometimes the very things we once saw as setbacks become the moments that shaped us the most. What looks like a detour in real time can turn out to be the exact path we needed to grow. Gratitude helps us hold both the beauty and the mess of life, and still find meaning in the middle.

THE HABIT OF GRATITUDE

Gratitude is a muscle. The more you use it, the more it grows. Here are a few ways to build a daily practice:

- Keep a gratitude journal. Write down three things you're thankful for – even small moments count.

- Send a message of thanks or simply think of someone who's helped you and silently offer them appreciation.

- Show it through small gestures: make someone a cup of tea, lend a hand or offer a genuine compliment.

- Revisit memories where someone showed you kindness and feel that moment again.

- Take a mindful pause to notice something in your environment – the light, a sound, the comfort of your chair – and acknowledge it with gratitude.

- Read or listen to something uplifting that helps you shift focus towards what's working.

- If you pray, let gratitude be your entry point.

- And when life feels heavy, ask: *What silver lining might be hidden here?* The lesson may not appear right away, but the willingness to look is a powerful start.

CHAPTER SUMMARY

Living with purpose is one of the most powerful things you can do for your health and longevity. Whether through journalling, meditation or simply paying closer attention to what brings you alive, self-reflection helps you reconnect with what matters most. The Japanese concept of ikigai – the intersection of what you love, what you're good at, what the world needs and what can sustain you – reminds us that purpose is not a destination but a direction. It's something you live into, one intentional choice at a time.

Surrounding yourself with people who truly see and support you is equally vital. Deep friendships and loving partnerships have been shown to reduce stress, boost resilience and even extend lifespans. Relationships give life meaning; not just through support but through shared joy, laughter and belonging. Even simple acts like caring for a pet, watering a plant or practising gratitude can offer powerful daily anchors to purpose and wellbeing.

Science continues to confirm what many ancient traditions already knew: joy, love, connection and meaning are biological. Laughter calms the nervous system. Gratitude lowers blood pressure. A sense of purpose strengthens immunity. The body listens to how you live.

So yes – take care of your health. But also: laugh more. Love deeply. Plant something. Dance often. And never underestimate the power of small moments lived with intention.

You don't have to wait to feel ready to begin. The future is shaped by how you live now, and the best time to start living young is today.

ACKNOWLEDGEMENTS

A very special thank you to Sergey Young, whose vision and passion for the pursuit of longevity have been a constant source of inspiration. An extraordinary mentor and trailblazer in the field of health and innovation, we are grateful for your support.

To Nadia, Sergey, Tim and Polina – for their unconditional love and unwavering support. Many things, including this book, would not have been possible without your encouragement.

To the Scicomwiz team, thank you for your talent, heart and dedication at every step. To Michelle – for your sharp eye, scientific rigor and care in shaping this book. And to our clients – the visionary experts who inspire us daily – this book is rooted in all we have learned from you.

To Nicki Crossley, Gabriella Nemeth, Lucy Stewardson, Lizzy Hey, Vicky Bywater and the entire team at Michael O'Mara Books – for believing in this project and helping bring it to life. Your guidance, expertise and support have been invaluable throughout this journey.

ABOUT THE AUTHORS

Dr Lara Hemeryck is a Belgian stem cell researcher and obtained her PhD in Biomedical Sciences from the University of Leuven. Lara founded science communication agency Scicomwiz, which specializes in health brands, longevity clinics and thought leaders. She has contributed as the lead researcher on multiple bestselling books, including *The Glucose Goddess Method* by Jessie Inchauspé, an instant *New York Times* bestseller.

Anastasia Mabel is part of the Sergey Young Foundation, one of the leading names in the longevity space. She specializes in health and longevity communications, shaped by her own recovery from a long-term chronic condition – an experience that fuels her commitment to making evidence-based wellness more accessible and actionable for all.

REFERENCES

EAT

Fadnes, L. T. et al. (2023). Life Expectancy Can Increase by up to 10 Years Following Sustained Shifts Towards Healthier Diets in the United Kingdom. *Nature Food*, 4:961–965. doi: 10.1038/s43016-023-00868-w

NHS (2022). The Eatwell Guide. *Public Health England.* https://www.nhs.uk/live-well/eat-well/food-guidelines-and-food-labels/the-eatwell-guide/ [last accessed 23 March 2025]

Shafqat, A. et al. (2024). Mediterranean Diet Adherence and Risk of All-Cause Mortality in Women. *JAMA Network Open.* doi: 10.1001/jamanetworkopen.2024.14322

Hughes, D. A. (1999). Effects of Carotenoids on Human Immune Function. *Proceedings of the Nutrition Society*, 58(3):713–718. doi: 10.1017/S0029665199000932

Johra, F. T. et al. (2020). A Mechanistic Review of β-Carotene, Lutein, and Zeaxanthin in Eye Health and Disease. *Antioxidants*, 9(11):1046. doi: 10.3390/antiox9111046

Wu, J. et al. (2015). Intakes of Lutein, Zeaxanthin, and Other Carotenoids and Age-Related Macular Degeneration During 2 Decades of Prospective Follow-up. *JAMA Ophthalmology*, 133(12):1415–1424. doi: 10.1001/jamaophthalmol.2015.3590

Rasmussen, H. M. et al. (2013). Nutrients for the Aging Eye. *Clinical Interventions in Aging*, 8:741–748. doi: 10.2147/CIA.S45399

Bondonno, C. P. et al. (2021). Vegetable Nitrate Intake, Blood Pressure and Incident Cardiovascular Disease: Danish Diet, Cancer, and Health Study. *European Journal of Epidemiology*, 36(8):813–825. doi: 10.1007/s10654-021-00747-3

Kapała, A. et al. (2022). The Anti-Cancer Activity of Lycopene: A Systematic Review of Human and Animal Studies. *Nutrients*, 14(23):5152. doi: 10.3390/nu14235152

Paul, R. et al. (2020). Lycopene – A Pleiotropic Neuroprotective Nutraceutical: Deciphering Its Therapeutic Potentials in Broad Spectrum Neurological Disorders. *Neurobiology of Aging*, 87:104823. doi: 10.1016/j.neuint.2020.104823

Unlu, N. Z. et al. (2007). Lycopene from Heat-Induced Cis-Isomer-Rich Tomato Sauce Is More Bioavailable Than from All-Trans-Rich Tomato Sauce in Human Subjects. *British Journal of Nutrition*, 98(1):140-146. doi: 10.1017/S0007114507685201

Sperber A. D. et al. (2021). Worldwide Prevalence and Burden of Functional Gastrointestinal Disorders, Results of Rome Foundation Global Study. *Gastroenterology*, 160(1):99-114. e3. doi: 10.1053/j.gastro.2020.04.014. Epub 2020 Apr 12. PMID: 32294476

Imamura, F. et al. (2016). Effects of Saturated Fat, Polyunsaturated Fat, Monounsaturated Fat, and Carbohydrate on Glucose-Insulin Homeostasis: A Systematic Review and Meta-analysis of Randomised Controlled Feeding Trials. *PLOS Medicine*, 13(7):e1002087. doi: 10.1371/journal.pmed.1002087

Bayram, S. Ş, Kızıltan G. (2024). The Role of Omega- 3 Polyunsaturated Fatty Acids in Diabetes Mellitus Management: A Narrative Review. *Current Nutrition Reports*, 13(3):527–551. doi: 10.1007/s13668-024-00561-9. Epub 2024 Jul 20. PMID: 39031306; PMCID: PMC11327211

Pelkman, C. L. et al. (2004). Effects of Moderate-Fat (From Monounsaturated Fat) and Low-Fat Weight-Loss Diets on the Serum Lipid Profile in Overweight and Obese Men and Women. *The American Journal of Clinical Nutrition*, 79(2):204–212. doi: 10.1093/ajcn/79.2.204

Mori, T. A. et al. (2004). Omega-3 Fatty Acids and Inflammation. *Current Atherosclerosis Reports*, 6:461–467. doi: 10.1007/s11883-004-0087-5

Cabo, J. et al. (2012). Omega-3 Fatty Acids and Blood Pressure. *British Journal of Nutrition*, 107(S2):S195–S200. doi: 10.1017/S0007114512001584

Kipp-Sinanis, E. (2011). Environmental Impact of Aquaculture: Wild-Caught vs. Farmed Fish. *ResearchGate*. https://www.researchgate.net/publication/324165259_Environmental_Impact_of_Aquaculture_Wild-Caught_vs_Farmed_Fish [last accessed 5 February 2025]

Rose, D. J. (2014). Impact of Whole Grains on The Gut Microbiota: The Next Frontier for Oats? *British Journal of Nutrition*, 112(S2):S44–S49. doi: 10.1017/S0007114514002244

Gross, L. S. et al. (2004). Increased Consumption of Refined Carbohydrates and The Epidemic of Type 2 Diabetes in the United States: An Ecologic Assessment. *The American Journal of Clinical Nutrition*, 79(5):774–779. doi: 10.1093/ajcn/79.5.774

Nijssen, K. M. R. et al. (2023). Longer-Term Mixed Nut Consumption Improves Brain Vascular Function and Memory: A Randomized, Controlled Crossover Trial in Older Adults. *Clinical Nutrition*, 42(7):1067–1075. doi: 10.1016/j.clnu.2023.05.025

de Souza R. G. M. et al. (2017). Nuts and Human Health Outcomes: A Systematic Review. *Nutrients*, 9(12):1311. doi: 10.3390/nu9121311

Aune, D. et al. (2016). Nut Consumption and Risk of Cardiovascular Disease, Total Cancer, All-Cause and Cause-Specific Mortality: A Systematic Review and Dose-Response Meta-Analysis of Prospective Studies. *BMC Medicine*, 14:207. doi: 10.1186/s12916-016-0730-3

NHS (2023). Lactose Intolerance. NHS. https://www.nhs.uk/conditions/lactose-intolerance [last accessed 23 March 2025]

Gargano, D. et al. (2021). Food Allergy and Intolerance: A Narrative Review on Nutritional Concerns. *Nutrients*, 13:1638. doi: 10.3390/nu13051638

Williams, S. C. P. (2024). Researchers Discover How Chronic Inflammation Worsens Heart Failure. *Medical Xpress*. https://medicalxpress.com/news/2024-10-chronic-inflammation-worsens-heart-failure.html [last accessed 16 November 2024]

Ellulu, M. S. et al. (2022). Clinical and Biological Risk Factors Associated with Inflammation in Patients With Type 2 Diabetes Mellitus. *BMC Endocrine Disorders*, 22:16. doi: 10.1186/s12902-021-00925-0

Xiang, Y. et al. (2023). The Role of Inflammation in Autoimmune Disease: A Therapeutic Target. *Frontiers in Immunology*, 14:1267091. doi: 10.3389/fimmu.2023.1267091

Seidelmann, S. et al. (2018). Dietary Carbohydrate Intake and Mortality: A Prospective Cohort Study and Meta-Analysis. *The Lancet Public Health*, 3(9):e419–e428. doi: 10.1016/S2468-2667(18)30135-X

Matsumoto, M. et al. (2023). Evaluation of Protein Requirements Using the Indicator Amino Acid Oxidation Method: A Scoping Review. *The Journal of Nutrition*, 153(12):3472–3489. doi: 10.1016/j.tjnut.2023.07.015

Brock, S. (2024). Protein Needs for Adults 50+. *Stanford Lifestyle Medicine*. https://longevity.stanford.edu/lifestyle/2024/01/23/protein-needs-for-adults-50/ [last accessed 16 November 2024]

Weigle, D. S. et al. (2005). A High-Protein Diet Induces Sustained Reductions in Appetite, Ad Libitum Caloric Intake, and Body Weight Despite Compensatory Changes in Diurnal Plasma Leptin And Ghrelin Concentrations. *American Journal of Clinical Nutrition*, 82(1):41–48. doi: 10.1093/ajcn.82.1.41

U.S. Centers for Disease Control and Prevention (2024). MTHFR Gene Variant and Folic Acid Facts. *U.S. Centers for Disease Control and Prevention*. https://www.cdc.gov/folic-acid/data-research/mthfr/index.html [last accessed 16 November 2024]

Anton, S. D. et al. (2018). Flipping the Metabolic Switch: Understanding and Applying the Health Benefits of Fasting. *Obesity (Silver Spring)*, 26(2):254–268. doi: 10.1002/oby.22065

Diab, R. et al. (2024). Intermittent Fasting Regulates Metabolic Homeostasis and Improves Cardiovascular Health. *Cell Biochemistry and Biophysics*, 82:1583–1597. doi: 10.1007/s12013-024-01314-9

Helfand, S. L. et al. (2021). Evidence That Overnight Fasting Could Extend Healthy Lifespan. *Nature*, 598:265–266. doi: 10.1038/d41586-021-01578-8

Roncal-Jimenez, C. et. al (2015). Mechanisms by Which Dehydration May Lead to Chronic Kidney Disease. *Annals of Nutrition and Metabolism*, 66 (Suppl. 3):10–13. doi: 10.1159/000381239

Scott, A. M. et al. (2020). Increased Fluid Intake to Prevent Urinary Tract Infections: Systematic Review And Meta-Analysis. *British Journal of General Practice*, 70(692):e200–e207. doi: 10.3399/bjgp20X708125

Burton, R. et al. (2018). No Level of Alcohol Consumption Improves Health. *The Lancet*, 392(10152):987–988. doi: 10.1016/S0140-6736(18)31571-X

The World Health Organization (2024). Alcohol. https://www.who.int/news-room/fact-sheets/detail/alcohol [last accessed 16 November 2024]

Valenzuela, C. F. (1997). Alcohol and Neurotransmitter Interactions. Alcohol Health and Research World, 21(2):144–148. https://pmc.ncbi.nlm.nih.gov/articles/PMC6826822/ [last accessed 16 November 2024]

Zhao, Y. et al. (2024). Association of Coffee Consumption and Prediagnostic Caffeine Metabolites with Incident Parkinson Disease in a Population-Based Cohort. *Neurology Journals*. doi: 10.1212/WNL.0000000000209201

Kunutsor S. K, Lehoczki A, Laukkanen J. A. (2025). Coffee consumption, cancer, and healthy aging: epidemiological evidence and underlying mechanisms. *GeroScience*, 47(2):1517-1555. doi: 10.1007/s11357-024-01332-8. Epub 2024 Sep 13. PMID: 39266809; PMCID: PMC11978573

Vigne, M. et al. (2023). Chronic Caffeine Consumption Curbs rTMS-Induced Plasticity. *Frontiers in Psychiatry*, 14:1137681. doi: 10.3389/fpsyt.2023.1137681

Bougrine, H. et al. (2024). Effects of Various Caffeine Doses on Cognitive Abilities in Female Athletes with Low Caffeine Consumption. *Brain Science*, 14(3):280. doi: 10.3390/brainsci14030280

Lovallo, W. R. et al. (2005). Caffeine Stimulation of Cortisol Secretion Across the Waking Hours in Relation to Caffeine Intake Levels. *Psychosomatic Medicine*, 67(5):734–739. doi: 10.1097/01.psy.0000181270.20036.06

O'Callaghan, F. et al. (2018). Effects of Caffeine on Sleep Quality and Daytime Functioning. *Risk Management and Healthcare Policy*, 11:263–271. doi: 10.2147/RMHP.S156404

Amer, S. A. et al. (2023). Caffeine Addiction and Determinants of Caffeine Consumption Among Health Care Providers: A Descriptive National Study. *European Review for Medical and Pharmacological Sciences*, 27(8):3230–3242. https://pubmed.ncbi.nlm.nih.gov/37140274/ [last accessed 16 November 2024]

Lyon, P. et al (2020). B Vitamins and One-Carbon Metabolism: Implications in Human Health and Disease. *Nutrients*, 12(9):2867. doi: 10.3390/nu12092867

Kovatcheva, M. et al. (2023). Vitamin B12 Is a Limiting Factor for Induced Cellular Plasticity and Tissue Repair. *Nature Metabolism*, 5:1911–1930. doi: 10.1038/s42255-023-00916-6

Field, D. T. et al. (2022). High-Dose Vitamin B6 Supplementation Reduces Anxiety and Strengthens Visual Surround Suppression. *Human Psychopharmacology: Clinical and Experimental*, 37(6):e2852. doi: 10.1002/hup.2852

Morris, M. S. et al. (2012). Vitamin B-12 and Folate Status in Relation to Decline in Scores on the Mini-Mental State Examination in the Framingham Heart Study. *Journal of the American Geriatrics Society*, 60:1457–1464. doi: 10.1111/j.1532-5415.2012.04076.x

Tardy, A.L. et al. (2020). Vitamins and Minerals for Energy, Fatigue and Cognition: A Narrative Review of the Biochemical and Clinical Evidence. *Nutrients*, 12(1):228. doi: 10.3390/nu12010228

Cashman, K. D. et al. (2016). Vitamin D Deficiency in Europe: Pandemic? *The American Journal of Clinical Nutrition*, 103(4):1033–1044. doi: 10.3945/ajcn.115.116978

Melrose, S. (2015). Seasonal Affective Disorder: An Overview of Assessment and Treatment Approaches. *Depression Research and Treatment*, 2015:178564. doi: 10.1155/2015/178564

National Institutes of Health (2022). Magnesium. Fact Sheet for Health Professionals. National Institutes of Health, Office of Dietary Supplements. https://ods.od.nih.gov/factsheets/Magnesium-HealthProfessional [last accessed 6 February 2025]

Vink, R. et al. (2011). Magnesium in the Central Nervous System [Internet]. Adelaide (AU): University of Adelaide Press; 2011. https://www.ncbi.nlm.nih.gov/books/NBK507264/ [last accessed 6 February 2025]

Yang, Y. et al. (2014). Alpha-Lipoic Acid Attenuates Insulin Resistance and Improves Glucose Metabolism In High Fat Diet-Fed Mice. *Acta Pharmacoliga Sinica*, 35(10):1285–1292. doi: 10.1038/aps.2014.64

Zhang, J. et al. (2023). Alpha Lipoic Acid Treatment in Late Middle Age Improves Cognitive Function: Proteomic Analysis of The Protective Mechanisms in The Hippocampus. *Neuroscience Letters*, 798:137098. doi: 10.1016/j.neulet.2023.137098

Rochette, L. et al. (2014). Alpha-Lipoic Acid – an Antioxidant with Protective Actions on Cardiovascular Diseases. In: Laher, I. (eds) *Systems Biology of Free Radicals and Antioxidants*, pp.1229–1249. Springer: Berlin, Heidelberg. doi: 10.1007/978-3-642-30018-9_77

Ma, G. P. et al. (2018). Rhodiola rosea L. Improves Learning and Memory Function: Preclinical Evidence and Possible Mechanisms. *Frontiers in Pharmacology*, 9:1415. doi: 10.3389/fphar.2018.01415

Lekomtseva, Y. et al. (2017). Rhodiola rosea in Subjects with Prolonged or Chronic Fatigue Symptoms: Results of an Open-Label Clinical Trial. *Complementary Medicine Research*, 24(1):46–52. doi: 10.1159/000457918

Igarashi, M. et al. (2022). Chronic nicotinamide mononucleotide supplementation elevates blood nicotinamide adenine dinucleotide levels and alters muscle function in healthy older men. *NPJ Aging*, 8(1):5. doi: 10.1038/s41514-022-00084-z. PMID: 35927255; PMCID: PMC9158788

Liao B. et al. (2021). Nicotinamide mononucleotide supplementation enhances aerobic capacity in amateur runners: a randomized, double-blind study. *Journal of the International Society of Sports*, 18(1):54.doi: 10.1186/s12970-021-00442-4. PMID: 34238308; PMCID: PMC8265078

Yoshino M. et al. (2021). Nicotinamide mononucleotide increases muscle insulin sensitivity in prediabetic women. *Science*, 372(6547):1224–1229. doi: 10.1126/science.abe9985. Epub 2021 Apr 22. PMID: 33888596; PMCID: PMC8550608

Rahman, S. U. et al. (2024). Role and Potential Mechanisms of Nicotinamide Mononucleotide in Aging. *Aging and Disease*, 15(2):565–583. doi: 10.14336/AD.2023.0519-1

Chak, K. C. et al. (2019). Pharmacological Basis and New Insights of Resveratrol Action in the Cardiovascular System. *British Journal of Pharmacology*. doi: 10.1111/bph.14801

Rodríguez-Enríquez, S. et al. (2019). Resveratrol Inhibits Cancer Cell Proliferation by Impairing Oxidative Phosphorylation and Inducing Oxidative Stress. *Toxicology and Applied Pharmacology*, 370:65–77. doi: 10.1016/j.taap.2019.03.008

Pyo, I. S. et al. (2020). Mechanisms of Aging and the Preventive Effects of Resveratrol on Age-Related Diseases. *Molecules*, 25(20):4649. doi: 10.3390/molecules25204649

Hsu, T. F. et al. (2021). Oral Hyaluronan Relieves Wrinkles and Improves Dry Skin: A 12-Week Double-Blinded, Placebo-Controlled Study. *Nutrients*, 13(7):2220. doi: 10.3390/nu13072220

Migliore, A. et al. (2015). Effectiveness and Utility of Hyaluronic Acid In Osteoarthritis. *Clinical Cases in Mineral and Bone Metabolism*, 12(1):31–33. doi: 10.11138/ccmbm/2015.12.1.031

Yousefzadeh, M. J. et al. (2018). Fisetin as a Senotherapeutic that Extends Health and Lifespan. *eBioMedicine*, 36:18–28. doi: 10.1016/j.ebiom.2018.09.015

Tavenier, J. et al. (2024). Fisetin as a senotherapeutic agent: Evidence and perspectives for age-related diseases, *Mechanisms of Ageing and Development*, 222:111995, ISSN 0047-6374

Lorenzo, E. C. et al. (2023). Impact of Senolytic Treatment on Immunity, Aging, and Disease. *Frontiers in Aging*, 4:1161799. doi: 10.3389/fragi.2023.1161799

Maher, P. (2024). The Flavonoid Fisetin Reduces Multiple Physiological Risk Factors for Dementia. *Neurochemistry International*, 178:105805. doi: 10.1016/j.neuint.2024.105805

Hofer, S. J. et al. (2002). Mechanisms of Spermidine-Induced Autophagy and Geroprotection. *Nature Aging* 2:1112–1129. doi: 10.1038/s43587-022-00322-9

Chen, Y. et al. (2021). Spermidine Affects Cardiac Function in Heart Failure Mice by Influencing the Gut Microbiota and Cardiac Galectin-3. *Frontiers in Cardiovascular Medicine*, 8:765591. doi: 10.3389/fcvm.2021.765591

Ni, Y. Q. et al. (2021). New Insights into the Roles and Mechanisms of Spermidine in Aging and Age-Related Diseases. *Aging and Disease*, 12(8):1948–1963. doi: 10.14336/AD.2021.0603

MOVE

Venkatasamy, V. V. et al. (2013). Effect of Physical Activity on Insulin Resistance, Inflammation and Oxidative Stress in Diabetes Mellitus. *Journal of Clinical and Diagnostic Research*, 7(8):1764–1766. doi: 10.7860/JCDR/2013/6518.3306

Guan, Y. et al. (2022). Molecular Mechanisms of Exercise and Healthspan. *Cells*, 11(5):872. doi: 10.3390/cells11050872

Anderson, E. et al. (2019). Physical Activity, Exercise, and Chronic Diseases: A Brief Review. *Sports Medicine and Health Science*, 1(1):3–10. doi: 10.1016/j.smhs.2019.08.006

Guan, Y. et al. (2022). Molecular Mechanisms of Exercise and Healthspan. *Cells*, 11(5):872. doi: 10.3390/cells11050872

Srikanthan P, Karlamangla AS. (2014). Muscle mass index as a predictor of longevity in older adults. *The American Journal of Medicine*, 127(6):547–553. doi: 10.1016/j.amjmed.2014.02.007. Epub 2014 Feb 18. PMID: 24561114; PMCID: PMC4035379

Geiger, C. et al. (2024). DNA Methylation of Exercise-Responsive Genes Differs Between Trained and Untrained Men. *BMC Biology*, 22(1):147. doi: 10.1186/s12915-024-01938-6

Dolezal, B. A. et al. (2017). Interrelationship between Sleep and Exercise: A Systematic Review. *Advances in Preventive Medicine*, 2017:1364387. doi: 10.1155/2017/1364387

Wolfe R. R. (2006). The underappreciated role of muscle in health and disease. *The American Journal of Clinical Nutrition*, 84(3):475–482. doi: 10.1093/ajcn/84.3.475. PMID: 16960159

Bohannon R. W. (2019). Grip Strength: An Indispensable Biomarker For Older Adults. *Clinical Interventions in Aging*, 14:1681–1691. doi: 10.2147/CIA.S194543. PMID: 31631989; PMCID: PMC6778477

Kim J. (2021). Handgrip Strength to Predict the Risk of All-Cause and Premature Mortality in Korean Adults: A 10-Year Cohort Study. *International Journal of Environmental Research and Public Health*, 19(1):39. doi: 10.3390/ijerph19010039. PMID: 35010298; PMCID: PMC8751337

Kemala Sari, N. et al. (2025). Handgrip strength as a potential indicator of aging: insights from its association with aging-related laboratory parameters. *Front Med* (Lausanne), 12:1491584. doi: 10.3389/fmed.2025.1491584. PMID: 39944493; PMCID: PMC11814436

Pinckard, K. et al. (2019). Effects of Exercise to Improve Cardiovascular Health. *Frontiers in Cardiovascular Medicine*, 6:69. doi: 10.3389/fcvm.2019.00069

Blondell, S. J. et al. (2014). Does Physical Activity Prevent Cognitive Decline And Dementia?: A Systematic Review and Meta-Analysis of Longitudinal Studies. *BMC Public Health*, 14:510. doi: 10.1186/1471-2458-14-510

Atakan, M. M. et al. (2021). Evidence-Based Effects of High-Intensity Interval Training on Exercise Capacity and Health: A Review with Historical Perspective. *International Journal of Environmental Research and Public Health*, 18(13):7201. doi: 10.3390/ijerph18137201

Stankovic, M. et al. (2023). Effects of High-Intensity Interval Training (HIIT) on Physical Performance in Female Team Sports: A Systematic Review. *Sports Medicine – Open* 9:78. doi: 10.1186/s40798-023-00623-2

Solan, M. (2024). Cognitive Benefits from High-Intensity Interval Training May Last for Years. Harvard Health Publishing. https://www.health.harvard.edu/exercise-and-fitness/cognitive-benefits-from-high-intensity-interval-training-may-last-for-years [last accessed 16 November 2024]

Nygaard H, Tomten SE, Høstmark AT. (2009). Slow postmeal walking reduces postprandial glycemia in middle-aged women. *Applied Physiology, Nutrition and Metabolism = Physiologie appliquée, nutrition et metabolisme*, 34(6):1087–1092.doi: 10.1139/H09-110. PMID: 20029518

Stens, N. A. et al. (2023). Relationship of Daily Step Counts to All-Cause Mortality and Cardiovascular Events. *Journal of the American College of Cardiology*, 82(15):1483–1494. doi: 10.1016/j.jacc.2023.07.029. Epub 2023 Sep 6. PMID: 37676198

Inoue, K. et al. (2023). Association of Daily Step Patterns With Mortality in US Adults. *JAMA Network Open*. 6(3):e235174. doi: 10.1001/jamanetworkopen.2023.5174. Erratum in: *JAMA Network Open*, 6(4):e2311413. doi: 10.1001/jamanetworkopen.2023.11413. PMID: 36976556; PMCID: PMC10051082

Sakuragi S, Sugiyama Y. (2006). Effects of daily walking on subjective symptoms, mood and autonomic nervous function. *Journal of Physiological Anthropology*, 25(4):281–289. doi: 10.2114/jpa2.25.281. PMID: 16891758

Oppezzo, M. et al. (2014). Give Your Ideas Some Legs: The Positive Effect of Walking on Creative Thinking. *Journal of Experimental Psychology: Learning, Memory, and Cognition*, 40(4):1142–1152. doi: 10.1037/a0036577

Li Q. (2010). Effect of forest bathing trips on human immune function. *Environmental Health and Preventative Medicine*, 15(1):9–17. doi: 10.1007/s12199-008-0068-3. PMID: 19568839; PMCID: PMC2793341

Talen, M. R. (2024). The Good Life: Lessons From the World's Longest Scientific Study of Happiness. *Family Medicine*, 56(10):684–685. doi: 10.22454/FamMed.2024.345850. PMCID: PMC11575524

NHS (2024). Physical Activity Guidelines for Adults Aged 19 to 64. NHS. https://www.nhs.uk/live-well/exercise/physical-activity-guidelines-for-adults-aged-19-to-64 [last accessed on 9 February 2024]

Dossett, M. L. et al (2020). A New Era for Mind–Body Medicine. *The New England Journal of Medicine*, 382:1390–1391. doi: 10.1056/NEJMp1917461

Nelson, S. et al. (2024). Biomarkers of Stress as Mind–Body Intervention Outcomes for Chronic Pain: An Evaluation of Constructs and Accepted Measurement. *PAIN* 165(11):2403–2408. doi: 10.1097/j.pain.0000000000003241

Skelly, A. et al. (2018). Non-invasive Nonpharmacological Treatment for Chronic Pain: A Systematic Review [Internet]. *Agency for Healthcare Research and Quality (US)*, Report No.: 18-EHC013-EF, PMID:30179389. https://pubmed.ncbi.nlm.nih.gov/30179389/ [last accessed 16 November 2024]

Cramer, H. et al. (2017). Effects Of Yoga on Chronic Neck Pain: A Systematic Review and Meta-Analysis. *Clinical Rehabilitation*, 31(11):1457–1465. doi: 10.1177/0269215517698735

Wang, Y. et al. (2018). Integrative Effect of Yoga Practice in Patients with Knee Arthritis: A PRISMA-Compliant Meta-Analysis. *Medicine (Baltimore)*, 97(31):e11742. doi: 10.1097/MD.0000000000011742

Gothe, N. P. et al. (2019). Yoga Effects on Brain Health: A Systematic Review of the Current Literature. *Brain Plasticity*, 5(1):105–122. doi: 10.3233/BPL-190084

Oh, B. et al. (2020). The Effects of Tai Chi and Qigong on Immune Responses: A Systematic Review and Meta-Analysis. *Medicines (Basel)*, 7(7):39. doi: 10.3390/medicines7070039

Wang, F. et al. (2013). The Effects of Qigong on Anxiety, Depression, and Psychological Well-Being: A Systematic Review and Meta-Analysis. *Evidence-Based Complementary Alternative Medicine*, 2013:152738. doi: 10.1155/2013/152738

Laukkanen, T. et al. (2018). Sauna bathing is associated with reduced cardiovascular mortality and improves risk prediction in men and women: a prospective cohort study. *BMC Medicine*, 16(1):219. doi: 10.1186/s12916-018-1198-0. PMID: 30486813; PMCID: PMC6262976

Huo, C. et al. (2022). Effect of Acute Cold Exposure on Energy Metabolism and Activity of Brown Adipose Tissue in Humans: A Systematic Review and Meta-Analysis. *Frontiers in Physiology*, 13:917084. doi: 10.3389/fphys.2022.917084

Yankouskaya, A. et al. (2023). Short-Term Head-Out Whole-Body Cold-Water Immersion Facilitates Positive Affect and Increases Interaction between Large-Scale Brain Networks. *Biology (Basel)*, 12(2):211. doi: 10.3390/biology12020211

Cain, T. et al. (2025). Effects of cold-water immersion on health and wellbeing: A systematic review and meta-analysis. *PLoS One*, 20(1):e0317615. doi: 10.1371/journal.pone.0317615. PMID: 39879231; PMCID: PMC11778651

Mullington, J. M. et al. (2009). Cardiovascular, inflammatory, and metabolic consequences of sleep deprivation. *Progress in Cardiovascular Diseases*, 51(4):294–302.doi: 10.1016/j.pcad.2008.10.003. PMID: 19110131; PMCID: PMC3403737

Irwin, M. R. et al. (1994). Partial sleep deprivation reduces natural killer cell activity in humans. *Psychosomatic Medicine*, 56(6):493–498

Potter, L.M. et al. (2015). Short Sleepers are Four Times More Likely to Catch a Cold. University of California San Francisco. https://www.ucsf.edu/news/2015/08/131411/short-sleepers-are-four-times-more-likely-catch-cold [last accessed 16 November 2024]

Sandhu A, Seth M, Gurm HS. (2014). Daylight savings time and myocardial infarction. *Open Heart*, 1(1):e000019. doi: 10.1136/openhrt-2013-000019. PMID: 25332784; PMCID: PMC4189320

SLEEP

National Institute on Aging (2020). A Good Night's Sleep. National Institute on Aging. https://www.nia.nih.gov/health/sleep/good-nights-sleep [last accessed 16 November 2024]

Casagrande, M. et al. (2022). Sleep Quality and Aging: A Systematic Review on Healthy Older People, Mild Cognitive Impairment and Alzheimer's Disease. *International Journal of Environmental Research and Public Health*, 19(14): 8457. doi: 10.3390/ijerph19148457

Gooley, J. J. et al. (2011). Exposure to room light before bedtime suppresses melatonin onset and shortens melatonin duration in humans. *The Journal of Clinical Endocrinology and Metabolism*, 96(3):E463–E472.doi: 10.1210/jc.2010-2098. Epub 2010 Dec 30. PMID: 21193540; PMCID: PMC3047226

Zaki, N. F. W. et al. (2020). Basic chronobiology: what do sleep physicians need to know? *Sleep Science*, 13(4):256–266. 13(4):256-266. doi: 10.5935/1984-0063.20200026. PMID: 33564373; PMCID: PMC7856659

Colrain I. M, Nicholas CL, Baker FC. (2014). Alcohol and the sleeping brain. *Handbook of Clinical Neurology*, 125:415–431.doi: 10.1016/B978-0-444-62619-6.00024-0. PMID: 25307588; PMCID: PMC5821259

Mullington, J. M. et al. (2010). Sleep loss and inflammation. *Best Practice & Research. Clinical Endocrinology & Metabolism*, 24(5):775–784. doi: 10.1016/j.beem.2010.08.014. PMID: 21112025; PMCID: PMC3548567

Doherty, R. et al. (2023). The Impact of Kiwifruit Consumption on the Sleep and Recovery of Elite Athletes. *Nutrients*, 15(10):2274. doi: 10.3390/nu15102274. PMID: 37242157; PMCID: PMC10220871

Diniz, G. et al. (2023). The effects of gratitude interventions: a systematic review and meta-analysis. *Einstein (Sao Paulo)*, 21:eRW0371. doi: 10.31744/einstein_journal/2023RW0371. PMID: 37585888; PMCID: PMC10393216

Wang X, Song C. (2023). The impact of gratitude interventions on patients with cardiovascular disease: a systematic review. *Frontiers in Psychology*, 14:1243598. doi: 10.3389/fpsyg.2023.1243598. PMID: 37809310; PMCID: PMC10551131

Liu, D. et al. (2023). Tumor Vaccines: Unleashing the Power of the Immune System to Fight Cancer. *Pharmaceuticals (Basel)*, 16(10):1384. doi: 10.3390/ph16101384

THINK

Kozlov, M. (2024). 'Mini Liver' Will Grow in Person's Own Lymph Node in Bold New Trial. Nature. https://www.nature.com/articles/d41586-024-00975-z [last accessed 15 November 2024]

Shaw, W. et al. (2024). Stress Effects on the Body. American Psychological Association. https://www.apa.org/topics/stress/body [last accessed 16 November 2024]

Vulcano, B.A. et al. (1984). The Prevalence of Psychosomatic Disorders Among a Sample of Police Officers. *Social Psychiatry*, 19:181–186. doi.org/10.1007/BF00596783

Li, Y. et al. (2020). Effects of Mindfulness Meditation on Anxiety, Depression, Stress, and Mindfulness in Nursing Students: A Meta-Analysis and Trial Sequential Analysis of Randomized Controlled Trials. *Frontiers of Nursing*, 7(1). doi: 10.2478/fon-2020-000

Marques, P. et al. (2018). Benefits of Mindfulness Meditation in Reducing Blood Pressure and Stress in Patients with Arterial Hypertension. *Journal of Human Hypertension*, 33:237–247. doi: 10.1038/s41371-018-0130-6

Santosa, I. et al. (2024). The effect of meditation on telomerase and stem cell. *International Journal of Research in Medical Sciences*, 12, 3491–3499. doi:10.18203/2320-6012. ijrms20242638

Black, D. S. et al. (2016). Mindfulness Meditation and The Immune System: A Systematic Review of Randomized Controlled Trials. *Annals of the New York Academy of Sciences*, 1373(1):13–24. doi: 10.1111/nyas.12998

Khoa, D. L. N. et al. (2019). Loving-Kindness Meditation Slows Biological Aging in Novices: Evidence from a 12-Week Randomized Controlled Trial. *Psychoneuroendocrinology*, 108:20–27. doi: 10.1016/j.psyneuen.2019.05.020

Bhasin, M.K. et al. (2018). Specific Transcriptome Changes Associated with Blood Pressure Reduction in Hypertensive Patients After Relaxation Response Training. *Journal of Alternative Complementary Medicine*, 24(5):486–504. doi: 10.1089/acm.2017.0053

Goyal, M. et al. (2014). Meditation Programs for Psychological Stress and Well-being: A Systematic Review and Meta-analysis. *JAMA Internal Medicine*, 174(3):357–368. doi: 10.1001/jamainternmed.2013.13018

Remskar, M. et al. (2024). Mindfulness Improves Psychological Health and Supports Health Behaviour Cognitions: Evidence From a Pragmatic RCT of a Digital Mindfulness-Based Intervention. *British Journal of Health Psychology*, 29(4). doi: 10.1111/bjhp.12745

Arco, A.D. et al. (2009). Neurotransmitters and Prefrontal Cortex–Limbic System Interactions: Implications for Plasticity and Psychiatric Disorders. *Journal of Neural Transmission*, 116:941–952. doi: 10.1007/s00702-009-0243-8

Waters, J. (2021). Constant Craving: How Digital Media Turned Us All into Dopamine Addicts. *Guardian*. https://www.theguardian.com/global/2021/aug/22/how-digital-media-turned-us-all-into-dopamine-addicts-and-what-we-can-do-to-break-the-cycle [last accessed 29 March 2025]

Ferreri, L. et al. (2019). Dopamine Modulates the Reward Experiences Elicited by Music. *Proceedings of the National Academy of Sciences of the United States of America*. doi: 10.1073/pnas.1811878116

Pauwels L. et al. (2018). Aging and Brain Plasticity. *Aging (Albany NY)*, 10(8):1789–1790. doi: 10.18632/aging.101514

Langer, E. J. (2009). Counterclockwise: Mindful Health and the Power of Possibility. Ballantine Books, New York

Levy, B. R. et al. (2022). Longevity Increased by Positive Self-perceptions of Aging. *Journal of Personality and Social Psychology*, 83(2):261–270. doi: 10.1037//0022-3514.83.2.261

Nakamura, J. S. et al. (2022). Associations Between Satisfaction with Aging and Health and Well-being Outcomes Among Older US Adults. *JAMA Network Open*, 5(2):e2147797. doi: 10.1001/jamanetworkopen.2021.47797

Tao Porchon-Lynch & Vard – Audition (America's Got Talent, 2015). YouTube. Uploaded by America's Got Talent 2015. https://www.youtube.com/watch?v=6YXnEwAUUkI [last accessed 14 February 2025]

Waxman, O. (2016). Grandma Moses Didn't Start Painting Until Her 70s. Here's Why. *TIME*. https://time.com/4482257/grandma-moses-history [last accessed 14 February 2025]

LIVE

Alimujiang, A. et al. (2019). Association Between Life Purpose and Mortality Among US Adults Older Than 50 Years. *JAMA Network Open*, 2(5):e194270. doi: 10.1001/jamanetworkopen.2019.4270

Witters, D. (2023). U.S. Depression Rates Reach New Highs. *Gallup*. https://news.gallup.com/poll/505745/depression-rates-reach-new-highs.aspx [last accessed 30 November 2024]

Mineo, L. (2017). Good Genes are Nice, but Joy is Better. *The Harvard Gazette*. https://news.harvard.edu/gazette/story/2017/04/over-nearly-80-years-harvard-study-has-been-showing-how-to-live-a-healthy-and-happy-life/ [last accessed 30 November 2024]

Lau, E. et al. (2014). Purpose-Driven Life: Life Goals as a Predictor of Quality of Life and Psychological Health. *Journal of Happiness Studies*, 16(5). doi: 10.1007/s10902-014-9552-1

Kim, E. S. et al. (2022). Sense of Purpose in Life and Subsequent Physical, Behavioral, and Psychosocial Health: An Outcome-Wide Approach. *American Journal of Health Promotion*, 36(1):137–147.doi: 10.1177/08901171211038545. Epub 2021 Aug 18. PMID: 34405718; PMCID: PMC8669210

Tanno, K. et al. (2009). Associations of Ikigai as a Positive Psychological Factor with All-Cause Mortality and Cause-Specific Mortality Among Middle-Aged and Elderly Japanese People: Findings from the Japan Collaborative Cohort Study. *Journal of Psychosomatic Research*, 67(1):67–75. doi: 10.1016/j.jpsychores.2008.10.018

Miyazaki, J. et al. (2022). Purpose in Life (Ikigai) and Employment Status in Relation to Cardiovascular Mortality: The Japan Collaborative Cohort Study. *BMJ Open*, 12:e059725. doi: 10.1136/bmjopen-2021-059725

World Economic Forum (2017). Is This Japanese Concept the Secret to a Long, Happy, Meaningful Life? World Economic Forum. https://www.weforum.org/stories/2017/08/is-this-japanese-concept-the-secret-to-a-long-life/ [last accessed 30 November 2024]

Grundström, J. et al. (2021). Associations Between Relationship Status and Mental Well-Being in Different Life Phases From Young to Middle Adulthood. *SSM – Population Health*, 14:100774. doi: 10.1016/j.ssmph.2021.100774

Wong, C. W. et al. (2019). Marital Status and Risk of Cardiovascular Diseases: a Systematic Review and Meta-Analysis. *Heart*, 104(23):1937–1948. doi: 10.1136/heartjnl-2018-313005

Schultz, W. et al. (2017). Marital Status and Outcomes in Patients with Cardiovascular Disease. *Journal of the American Heart Association*, 6(12). doi: 10.1161/JAHA.117.005890

Whisman, M. A. et al. (2018). Marital Satisfaction and Mortality in the United States Adult Population. *Health Psychology*, 37(11):1041–1044. doi: 10.1037/hea0000677

Neumann, I. D. (2007). Oxytocin: The Neuropeptide of Love Reveals Some of its Secrets. *Cell Metabolism*, 5(4):231–233. doi: 10.1016/j.cmet.2007.03.002

Benameur, T. et al. (2021). The Antiaging Role of Oxytocin. *Neural Regeneration Research*, 16(12):2413–2414. doi: 10.4103/1673-5374.313030

Monin, J. K. et al. (2011). Why Do Men Benefit More from Marriage Than Do Women? Thinking More Broadly About Interpersonal Processes That Occur Within and Outside of Marriage. *ResearchGate*. doi: 10.1007/s11199-011-0008-3

Holt-Lunstad, J. et al. (2010). Social Relationships and Mortality Risk: A Meta-analytic Review. *PLoS Medicine*. doi: 10.1371/journal.pmed.1000316

Office of the U.S. Surgeon General (2023). Our Epidemic of Loneliness and Isolation. https://www.hhs.gov/sites/default/files/surgeon-general-social-connection-advisory.pdf [last accessed 7 December 2024]

University of Maryland (2024). New Research Reveals Linkages Between Volunteerism & Social Connections. University of Maryland, School of Public Policy. https://dogood.umd.edu/news/new-research-reveals-linkages-between-volunteerism-social-connections-0 [last accessed 14 February 2025]

Hall, J. (2019). How Many Hours Does it Take to Make a Friend? *Journal of Social and Personal Relationships*, 36(4):1278–1296. doi: 10.1177/0265407518761225

Clower, T. L. et al. (2015). The Health Care Cost Savings of Pet Ownership. Human Animal Bond Research Initiative (HABRI) Foundation. https://habri.org/assets/uploads/HABRI_Report_-_Healthcare_Cost_Savings_from_Pet_Ownership_.pdf [last accessed 7 December 2024]

Kogan, L. R. et al. (2024). Dog Ownership and Survival: A Systematic Review and Meta-Analysis. *American Heart Association Journals*. doi: 10.3390/pets1020012

UC Davis Health (2024). Health Benefits of Pets: How Your Furry Friend Improves Your Mental And Physical Health. https://health.ucdavis.edu/blog/cultivating-health/health-benefits-of-pets-how-your-furry-friend-improves-your-mental-and-physical-health/2024/04 [last accessed 7 December 2024]

Clements, H. et al. (2019). The Effects of Interacting with Fish in Aquariums on Human Health and Well-Being: A Systematic Review. PLoS One, 14(7):e0220524. doi: 10.1371/journal.pone.0220524

Yahoo! News (2024). The Five Best Indoor Plants for a Better Night's Sleep. Yahoo News UK. https://uk.news.yahoo.com/five-best-indoor-plants-better-121235788.html [last accessed 30 March 2025]

Wolverton, B. C. et al. (1989). Interior Landscape Plants for Indoor Air Pollution Abatement. *NASA*. https://ntrs.nasa.gov/citations/19930073077 [last accessed 30 March 2025]

Han, K. T. et al. (2022). Effects of Indoor Plants on Human Functions: A Systematic Review with Meta-Analyses. *International Journal of Environmental Research and Public Health*, 19(12):7454. doi: 10.3390/ijerph19127454

Lee, M. et al. (2015). Interaction with Indoor Plants May Reduce Psychological and Physiological Stress by Suppressing Autonomic Nervous System Activity in Young Adults: A Randomized Crossover Study. *Journal of Physiological Anthropology*, 34:21. doi: 10.1186/s40101-015-0060-8

Nieuwenhuis, M. et al. (2014). The Relative Benefits of Green Versus Lean Office Space: Three Field Experiments. *Journal of Experimental Psychology: Applied*, 20(3):199–214. doi: 10.1037/xap0000024

Sakurada, K. et al. (2020). Associations of Frequency of Laughter with Risk of All-Cause Mortality and Cardiovascular Disease Incidence in a General Population: Findings From the Yamagata Study. *Journal of Epidemiology*, 30(4):188–193. doi: 10.2188/jea.JE20180249

Kim, J. (2007). Differences in Longevity Factors amongst Korean Centenarians, Octogenarians, and Sexagenarians. *Journal of Health Education and Promotion*, 24(5):55–68

Kramer, C. K. et al. (2023). Laughter As Medicine: A Systematic Review and Meta-Analysis of Interventional Studies Evaluating the Impact of Spontaneous Laughter on Cortisol Levels. *PLoS One*, 18(5):e0286260. doi: 10.1371/journal.pone.0286260

Manninen, S. et al. (2017). Social Laughter Triggers Endogenous Opioid Release in Humans. *Journal of Neuroscience*, 37(25):6125–6131. doi: 10.1523/JNEUROSCI.0688-16.2017

Miller, M. (2009). The Effect of Mirthful Laughter on the Human Cardiovascular System. *Medical Hypotheses*, 73(5):636–639. doi: 10.1016/j.mehy.2009.02.044

Chen, Y. et al. (2024). Gratitude and Mortality Among Older US Female Nurses. *JAMA Psychiatry*, 81(10):1030–1038. doi: 10.1001/jamapsychiatry.2024.1687

Harvard Health Publishing (2021). Giving Thanks Can Make You Happier. https://www.health.harvard.edu/healthbeat/giving-thanks-can-make-you-happier [last accessed 11 December 2024]

Jackowska, M. et al. (2015). The Impact of a Brief Gratitude Intervention on Subjective Well-Being, Biology and Sleep. *Journal of Health Psychology*, 21(10):2207–2217. doi: 10.1177/1359105315572455